D1566199

Lucy Jane King

From Under the Cloud
At Seven Steeples

1878-1885

The Peculiarly Saddened Life of Anna Agnew
at the Indiana Hospital for the Insane

Lucy Jane King, M.D.

Guild Press/Emmis Publishing, LP
Zionsville, IN

Cover credit: John Zwara, Watercolor, Indiana Medical History Museum
Back cover: Portrait of Anna Agnew, Indiana Historical Society

ISBN: 1-57860-106-1

Library of Congress Card No. 2002101456

Dedication

To the memory of Anna Agnew—

Who wanted to end misunderstanding, stigmatization, and abuse
of patients with psychiatric illnesses—

With the hope that her objective in writing a book in 1886
might someday be fully achieved—

Table of Contents

Preface

When I began work at the History of Medicine Collection, Ruth Lilly Medical Library, Indiana University School of Medicine, Nancy Eckerman, Special Collections Librarian, called my attention to *From under the Cloud* written in 1886 by Anna Agnew. Mrs. Eckerman, genealogy researcher Lynne Orvis, and I read the book and wanted to know more about the candid, literate author and the context in which she had lived. Fortunately, Anna Agnew had provided some clues. She had told us the name of her hometown and had referred to a few relatives by their first names.

The genealogical resources in Clermont County, Ohio, the original home of Anna Keyt Agnew and her family, have been of enormous help, including the Clermont County Probate Court Records Division and the Clermont County Public Library Genealogy Section, both in Batavia, Ohio. Billie Broadus, Director, Cincinnati Medical Heritage Museum and Library, University of Cincinnati School of Medicine, provided information about Anna Agnew's half-brother, Dr. Alonzo Keyt, and his family.

The Nineteenth Century Indiana Physician Biographies compiled by Nancy Eckerman and Lynne Orvis made it possible to detail the lives of physicians mentioned by Anna Agnew. I am especially indebted to Mrs. Eckerman, who introduced me to Anna Agnew's book, contributed her extensive knowledge of resources about the nineteenth century and the Civil War, and was always available to search out the most obscure reference. Lynne Orvis traveled with me to small towns, libraries, government offices, and cemeteries in Indiana and Ohio and graciously and generously shared her broad knowledge of genealogy and the use of genealogical resources.

Very special thanks are due Nancy Niblack Baxter of Guild Press/ Emmis Publishing, LP for her extensive and insightful editorial comments that provided an antidote to pedantry and polemics.

Lucy Jane King
Indiana University School of Medicine
Indianapolis
January 2002

Introduction

In 1886 Anna Agnew wrote a poignant history of her seven years at the Indiana Hospital for the Insane, *From under the Cloud*. Her experiences in the hospital and the surrounding events of her life had transformed her from the wife of a railroad clerk and mother of three into an author of nineteenth-century reform literature. Her book is unique in that it gives everyday details and a complete picture of life in an asylum.

This fascinating, well-written account describes the difficulties of experiencing an episodic illness, manic-depressive disease, which had to run its course because there were no effective treatments at the time. Severe psychiatric illness, in the context of the social and legal status of women in nineteenth-century America, cost Anna Agnew her marriage and the right to see her three children.

Typical of most people in the nineteenth-century, Mrs. Agnew's family physicians and her husband did not understand her illness. They simply did not realize what she was experiencing. Once patients were admitted to asylums for the insane, treatments varied, sometimes being humane, sometimes not.

Insanity has plagued individuals since the earliest times. Institutions to house the "mad" have been around for a thousand years. In Colonial America sufferers were derided, mocked, feared, and cast out; but by 1800 society in the new republic generally accepted that those with mental illness should be removed from the stresses of life and treated according to current medical theories.

Land had been set aside in Indianapolis in 1827 for a state hospital and lunatic asylum, but the institution was not built at that time. Instead, a log cabin was used as a "crazy house." An act of the Indiana legislature of 1844-45 provided for the erection of a State Lunatic Asylum. Construction was begun in 1846, and the first patients were admitted in 1848.

When Anna Agnew was admitted to the hospital in 1878 there were 614 patients in the hospital, a number exceeding that of any former year. By her last year as a patient there were 1,454 patients, and a new women's building had been added. This increase in patient load was due to industrialization and the concentration of people in cities.

The Indiana Hospital for the Insane, later called the Central State Hospital, went through cycles typical of many large public institutions. Superintendents, patients, politicians, and families complained to governors and legislators about deplorable conditions and patient abuse. Committees were appointed to investigate, monies were appropriated, new staffs were hired, and reforms were made. Eventually conditions deteriorated, and the cycle repeated. With Dickensian drama, Anna Agnew described the results in her own time.

The book provided vignettes of several superintendents of the Indiana Hospital for the Insane. In 1896 Superintendent Dr. George F. Edenharter opened a laboratory building for bacteriologic, microscopic, and pathologic study of mental disease, only the second American institution to continue the work of medical scientists in Europe studying psychiatric illness. The Pathological Department of the Central Indiana Hospital for the Insane that Dr. Edenharter opened now houses the Indiana Medical History Museum. Anna Agnew, her fellow patients, her doctors, and their staffs are part of that history.

Anna Agnew can educate us today. She described in striking detail the experience of untreated extreme mood swings, hallucinations, and suicide attempts and urged families to seek care for loved ones who needed it. She courageously spoke out against the stigmatization of "insanity." Her message is even more pertinent now that treatment is available but underutilized.

PART ONE

CHAPTER ONE

*A*sylum and Moral Treatment

They traveled through groves of natural forest trees beginning to turn bright autumn hues, past ornamental gardens and fountains. They had come eighty miles from Vincennes, Indiana from which they departed on September 26, 1878. Anna Agnew was forty-two years old and the mother of three young boys.

On October 5, 1878, the *Weekly Western Sun* in Vincennes, Indiana, reported: "A commission *de lunatico inquirendo* composed of J. H. Massey and Charles Heidenreich, Justices, were appointed last week to investigate the charges of insanity against Mrs. Annie Agnew, a resident of the eastern portion of the city. The affidavits state that symptoms of insanity have been shown for the past thirteen months, and that it reached a culminating point a short time ago when she administered an ounce of laudanum to her child, but without fatal effect. Upon application she was admitted to the State Insane Asylum, and was taken thence last Thursday, where, it is hoped, a speedy cure will be affected."

Hospital admitting records noted as "propensities" that she was "suicidal and homicidal." Anna Agnew had made several attempts on her life with overdoses of medication. State law in 1878 provided that after a respectable citizen had filed appropriate papers alleging insanity, an associate judge of the county, with assistance of a respectable physician, would visit and examine the allegedly insane person and make a declaration as to the person's sanity. If the judge declared the individual insane, the physician then made arrangements for admission to the Indiana Hospital for the Insane in Indianapolis.

The drama involved David Agnew, frustrated by his wife's severe illness that he could not understand; Anna Agnew, who was psychotically depressed; two judges; and the doctor who certified her insanity. Anna's illness was to have serious consequences not only for David and Anna, but also for their three little boys who had defended their mother's strange behavior to their playmates and were now on the point of losing her forever.

Anna Agnew later wrote:

> My first night spent at the asylum was a dreadful one to me although my attendants were very considerate to me. I was placed in a sleeping room in the receiving ward together with three other patients and immediately asked permission of Dr. [William W.] Hester to sleep in a room by myself since I was afraid of insane people. This request he refused assuring me that I had no more reason to be afraid of those other three insane women than they had to be afraid of me, a fact I certainly had not thought of before. But this was said kindly, and at bedtime he came in with the night watch explaining her duties and telling me the use of her little lantern, saying she would look in upon me frequently during the night, and I must not be frightened as she flashed her light into my face to see if I were sleeping. From that night I have loved that night watch and during the few months she remained there afterwards she was a friend indeed, as are all who are friends in need, and we are still friends and often since my recovery have talked over the sad hours of my affliction; and the ladies who have at different times since filled this responsible position during my stay there deserve unstinted praise for the punctual, watchful discharge of their lonely and sometimes fearful duties; for in the silent watches of the night these young girls are sometimes called upon to witness death in its most fearful form— self-inflicted! And to me in my years of almost entire sleeplessness they seemed by the glancing light of their lanterns as they flitted

Seven Steeples

"Seven Steeples," where Anna Agnew spent most of her years at the Indiana Hospital for the Insane, was the Department for Women, the building which had eight steeples. Legend had it that only seven steeples could be seen from any given point along the road outside the grounds. The four-story building had a thousand rooms. Large windows provided light and air. Located on spacious grounds in a grove of old forest trees, it was seen as a place that would provide restful asylum from the cares of the world.

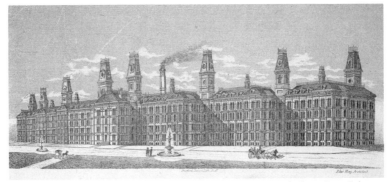

Indiana State Library

In the twentieth century Seven Steeples, which was opened while Anna Agnew was a patient in the late 1870s, became the main building of the hospital. In 1974, almost a century after it was first built, it too was demolished. By then modern cottages housed the patients.

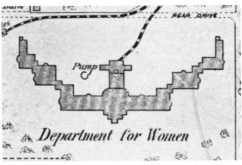

Indiana Medical History Museum

along with almost noiseless step like guardian spirits. I don't know that they even dreamed I loved them even when I appeared to be the reincarnation of hatefulness. I am glad of the opportunity of speaking thus publicly of their faithfulness to the trust placed in them.

Before I had been an inmate of the asylum a week I felt a greater degree of contentment than I had felt for a year previous. Not that I was reconciled to life, but because my unhappy condition of mind was understood, and I was treated accordingly. Besides, I was surrounded by others in like bewildered, discontented mental state in whose miseries, each believing their own individual woe the greater, I found myself becoming interested, my sympathies becoming aroused. I had always loved books but strangely enough had never read anything of insanity, had never thought but little about it, hence these insane people were a study—an interesting study, too.

And at the same time, I too, was treated as an insane woman, a kindness hitherto not shown me, Dr. Hester being the first person kind enough to say to me in answer to my question, "Am I insane?" "Yes, madam, and very insane, too! So much so that I very greatly doubt your recovery; and I must say further that had not the mistaken kindness of your friends kept you out of this place almost three years, you might now be at home a well woman with your children.

"But," he continued, "we intend to benefit you all we can and our particular hope for you is the restraint of this place." The insane have no better friend than Dr. Hester. I heard him once, in reprimanding a negligent attendant, give utterance to this noble sentiment: "I stand pledged to the State of Indiana to protect these unfortunates. I am the father, son, brother, and husband of over three hundred women!—a tolerably big contract—but I have undertaken it, and I'll see that they are well taken care of!"

Newly admitted patients often feel better after a few days of adjustment to the hospital. They no longer have to face the responsibilities that their illnesses prevented them from being able to meet. This was initially the idea of "asylum."

The recognition of Anna Agnew's illness for what it was reassured her. Neither her doctors at home nor her husband had recognized the nature of her disorder. Most people in the nineteenth century would have misunderstood her condition.

Theory: Moral Treatment

Insanity in women is obviously related to their ardent and nervous temperament, or so thought physicians in the nineteenth century, including Anna Agnew's physicians in Vincennes, Indiana. Women and the insane were characterized as being dependent, unable to govern themselves, and unable to direct their energies. The insane woman was in double jeopardy for restrictive measures. Menstrual cycles and female reproductive function clearly seemed to these mostly male doctors to be a cause of women's emotional states and nervous disorders.

The printed admission form for women patients at the Indiana Hospital for the Insane asked specifically: "Does the patient menstruate regularly, or is there disorder?" "Has the patient ovarian, uterine disease or displacement?" and "Specify symptoms and causes of present bodily infirmity," including all the rest of the organs under one question. Anna Agnew's admission form is filled in only for the first question: "Menses reported regular during past 5 or 6 mos.— prior-irregular."

We know now that women are more likely than men to suffer from major depressive disorder and panic disorder, while men are more likely to suffer from alcohol dependence and other substance dependence. Several other psychiatric disorders, including the bipolar disorder ("manic-depressive disease") experienced by Anna

Agnew, are experienced by equal numbers of men and women. Some women are more likely to have episodes of illness postpartum and other women experience premenstrual worsening of symptoms. But to this day a one-to-one link between female hormone function and psychiatric disorders in women has not been found.

Dr. Hester had been working with insane patients for more than a decade; his treatment reflected some of the ideas of psychiatric diagnosis in the first three quarters of the nineteenth century. He felt that if Anna Agnew had been treated early in her illness, recovery would have been likely. There were some data at the time suggesting that patients who had not been ill for long before admission were more likely to recover than those who had been ill for some years. This does not necessarily prove that early hospitalization prevents chronic disease. Perhaps many just had brief episodes of illness.

The year Anna Agnew was admitted to the Indiana Hospital for the Insane there were 614 patients at the beginning of the year; 470 were admitted; 470 patients were discharged: 273, recovered; 62, improved; 72, not improved; 4, not insane; and 59, died. At the end of the year 614 patients remained, 312 men and 302 women.

One study of thirty-nine American asylums in the 1800s by Pliny Earle, a well-known psychiatrist at the time, showed that there were more than 33,000 admissions and well over 9,000 patients discharged as recovered in a three-to-six-year period. This seems to reflect a recovery rate of about 30 percent. However, the admissions and discharges were not necessarily the *same* patients. As was the case for statistics reported for the Indiana Hospital for the Insane, the data do not take into account how long the admitted patients would stay in the hospital or how long the discharged patients had been there. The kinds of data available to Dr. Hester were incomplete and often statistically flawed.

Hester's faith in contemporary treatments was also based on the untested assumption that the treatments used made a difference in long-term outcome. That probably would not have been the case very frequently in psychiatry until the mid-twentieth century. Earlier hospitalization would, however, have prevented some of the devastating family problems resulting from Anna Agnew's illness and a series of serious suicide attempts that she made in the months prior to admission.

If a patient recovered, improvement was attributed to whatever treatment had been employed. Then, as now, the possibility was not always considered that some disorders characteristically have remissions. A fortunate physician takes over a case when the patient is getting better for whatever reason. Dr. Hester was not so fortunate. Anna Agnew would not experience improvement of her illness for six years.

Dr. William W. Hester was Anna Agnew's physician during the first nine months of her hospitalization. Born in southern Indiana not far from Louisville, Kentucky, he had served in the 3rd. Kentucky Cavalry of the Union forces during the Civil War. Before the war he had read medicine with a physician in Indiana and later graduated from Jefferson Medical College in Philadelphia. He was an assistant physician at the Indiana Hospital for the Insane from 1865 to 1879 and served in the same capacity at the Southern Hospital for the Insane, Anna, Illinois, from 1879 until 1890. For the remainder of his career he was in private practice in Chicago.

Anna Agnew continued her account:

This subject of restraint as a curative in the treatment of the insane was brought before me in a conversation with our superintendent, Dr. Orpheus Everts, a gentleman of superior attainments and experience and in whom centered all the virtues constituting the true philanthropist. I was one day standing as I frequently did at the window, sunken in the deepest melancholy, gazing at I know not what, when I was aroused by his voice asking, "Are you drinking in the beauties of nature ?" And truly the view from that point was lovely! But I answered, "I am not thinking at all whether the sun is shining or clouded; but I remember when I delighted in the loveliness of nature." "And you will again," he said. "Surely as the sun comes from behind the cloud, just so surely will you come from under the cloud now enveloping you." I thought differently, and said, "Upon what grounds do you base your hope for me?" "Principally, I think upon the restraint you are under in this place."

Dr. Everts had unwittingly given Anna Agnew the title of the book she would later write, *From under the Cloud*. His view of her prognosis seems somewhat more optimistic than that of Dr. Hester. Everts went on to point out that she could not escape from the barred windows and that she would be carried to eat and to bed if necessary. He noted that this would no doubt be difficult to one of her temperament. His comments referred both to concepts of the causes of mental illness and to ideas about treatment.

Prior to the late nineteenth century "madness" or "insanity" was seen as a single entity. A prominent American psychiatrist in the mid–nineteenth century wrote a paper defining insanity as "a chronic disease of the brain, producing either derangement of the intellectual faculties, or prolonged change of the feelings, affections, and habits of an individual." Many current day diagnoses representing different kinds of psychiatric disorders are covered by this definition. Not all are chronic.

Quiet, retarded patients were said to have melancholia; agitated patients, mania. Although some patients did have severe depression (melancholia) or mania, many diagnoses now used were included in these categories. That true mania and depression might succeed each other contributed to the idea that there was only one psychiatric illness, manifesting itself in different forms in different patients or at different times in the same patient.

Until late in the nineteenth century, illness was vaguely defined and seen as representing various imbalances of bodily processes. This concept can be traced to Hippocrates, that the balance of four "humors," or bodily fluids, determined disease. Understanding of body chemistry had, of course, become more sophisticated by the eighteenth century, but earlier presumptions about illness influenced the practice of medicine. A related idea prevalent at the time was that illness was controlled by temperament. As medical historian John Harley Warner has described, each temperament was associated with its characteristic behavior and required a specific therapeutic approach such as bleeding for the sanguine and cheerful, or purging for the choleric and hot tempered. An active temperament like that of Anna Agnew must be restrained as a part of treatment.

Historian Norman Dain has listed postulated causes in the nineteenth century for "insanity" like Anna's: family history, poor upbringing, sedentary life, febrile disease, overly pessimistic or overly optimistic view of life, ill-founded dread of divine vengeance, climate, and the government or economic system. Precipitating causes immediately preceding the illness included bodily disease, brain trauma, immoderate manual labor, excessive mental effort, masturbation, and strong emotion such as disappointment in love, business, or politics, or excessive pride, terror, or joy. Obviously, these causes are vague and contradictory. Any human being as well as any specific patient would have experienced several of them in any given year. Some of them might even represent results of psychiatric illness rather than causes.

In terms of treatment, asylums initially were conceived as places of respite from the stresses of the world. Philippe Pinel in France devised "Traitement Morale" in the eighteenth century to provide structure in such a setting. This "Moral Treatment" replaced bleeding, purging, massive sedation, and similar measures that characterized much of earlier medicine and employed ideas that would later become prominent in twentieth-century psychosocial treatments in psychiatric hospitals.

The restful and structured environment with regular schedules that asylums afforded was intended to help patients regain self-control. Kindly treatment of patients was emphasized. Employment in activities of daily living in the hospital, such as housekeeping and sewing, and interesting educational, recreational, and social activities were an integral part of the treatment. Severely ill patients were housed in different settings from those who were improving, allowing for the reward of moving to a more comfortable environment as improvement in symptoms occurred. Patients were encouraged to examine their lives and behaviors in an early version of what would later develop as psychologically sophisticated cognitive-behavioral therapy in the twentieth century.

And so, Anna benefited (though irregularly) from "moral treatment" of the insane. Everts's successor as superintendent, Dr. Joseph Rogers, who was superintendent during most of Anna Agnew's hospitalization, wrote of moral therapy:

> As regards moral treatment, no attempts are made to coax or force minds to act normally as long as the machine that thinks is in need of repair. When the material brain is restored to health, then its mysterious immaterial workings will be normal, and not till then. Pleasant social and material surroundings are necessary to general well being, and every effort is made to secure such as far as circumstances allow. Outdoor walks in pleasant weather, a little work for both men and women, when willing and able, amusements of various kinds in wards and elsewhere, books and journals; these are the distractions at present afforded, and efforts are being made to vary these still further. Several of the clergymen of Indianapolis have kindly offered to conduct quiet religious services with short homilies in the chapel whenever called upon. A dramatic and musical club has been organized, and have presented very praiseworthy amusements for both attendants and patients. A ten-pin alley and billiard-room are among the contemplated additions for this purpose. In short, no effort will be spared to make the residence agreeable to those whose faculties are only disturbed, and to afford awakening influences for those who have eyes but see not, and have ears but hear

not.

Even the architecture of the asylum was seen as important for moral therapy. Sites were selected outside a populated urban area, but they were accessible by roads and trains. A pleasing site and physical plant exerted a beneficial influence on patients. Good drainage and abundant water supply enhanced health while sufficient land provided outdoor exercise and agricultural activity. Beautiful in form, Seven Steeples was planned to exert a "beneficial influence" on patients.

Thomas Kirkbride, superintendent of the Pennsylvania Hospital for the Insane in Philadelphia, popularized these ideas in his writings. At his hospital, a central administrative building with wings on each side, one for female patients and one for male, gave a sense of graceful proportions to the structure. The front of the building was cut stone ornamented with a handsome Doric portico, spacious arched halls, and windows arranged for free circulation of air and light.

Kirkbride wrote a textbook about all aspects of construction, construction materials, food preparation, water supplies, sewers, and all other physical aspects of building and maintaining hospitals for the insane. He outlined the administrative organization in detail and discussed insanity and its treatment. He said the staff should include a superintendent physician who resided upon the premises, directing the medical, moral, and dietetic treatment and selecting other employees; an assistant physician who prepared and dispensed medication and supervised patient care; supervisors, one for each sex, to work among patients, to see that attendants were following the rules, and to prepare a written report for the physician each night of the days happenings.

"Seven Steeples," where Anna Agnew was housed, and the administrative organization of those who took care of her at the Indiana Hospital for the Insane followed Kirkbride's plans. When the new hospital was constructed in the 1840s to replace the original log cabin "crazy house," it was located two miles outside Indianapolis with ornamental gardens on the grounds and a small farm nearby to supply food for the hospital as well as useful activity for patients.

The experience of the hospital community was under the guidance of hospital superintendents, increasingly required to be physicians as the nineteenth century progressed and the medicalization of psychiatry developed. Founded in 1844, the Association of Medical Superintendents of American Institutions for the Insane was a forerunner of the current American Psychiatric Association and the first medical specialty society in this country. However, no specific requirements beyond the basic medical training of the day were required of superintendents. Specialization was acquired by experience in asylums, not by postgraduate training as in psychiatry residencies today.

Like many of his contemporaries Dr. Orpheus Everts had received medical training, often a matter of months to a year or two, from several sources. He was graduated from the Medical College of Indiana, LaPorte, in 1846; from the Medical Department of Michigan University in 1865; and from Rush Medical College, Chicago, in 1867. He was a surgeon in the 20th Indiana Infantry during the Civil War and superintendent of the Indiana Hospital for the Insane from 1868-79. He then became an asylum superintendent in Cincinnati.

Anna Agnew's reference to him as "a gentleman of superior attainment and experience" refers to his having written medical books and several volumes of poetry. After she had been discharged from the hospital, she visited Cincinnati and wrote in a letter, "One of the pleasantest features of my trip to Ohio was the privilege of spending part of a day with Dr. and Mrs. Everts at the Sanitarium at College Hill."

In talking to Anna Agnew, Dr. Everts had been referring to the structured schedules and the imposition of firm but kindly discipline that moral treatment employed. It did not include punitive, cruelly applied measures. Tragically, with population growth and urbanization, public institutions were required to take in larger and larger numbers of patients and often had too many patients and too few staff to make it possible to utilize the principles of moral treatment. Return to sedation (chemical restraint) and the use of harsh physical restraint seemed inevitable. The dream of enlightened moral therapy was difficult to realize.

Reality: Anna Agnew's Experience

A major problem was that the ideals of moral treatment espoused by these physicians were not always utilized in the wards when doctors were not there and control of the patients was in the hands of inadequately trained, in some cases cruel, attendants. Anna Agnew described vividly her experiences:

> I can truthfully say that there never was a time, subsequent, when I would not have obeyed a polite request. But unfortunately politeness is a virtue made conspicuous by its scarcity among attendants upon the insane, as many an indignant woman can testify. Generally they are of a class who use their brief authority to outrage and humiliate in every possible manner the persons so unfortunate as to be in their power.
>
> Certainly the position of an attendant upon the insane is not an agreeable one—at times it is extremely unpleasant—but it is not compulsory upon these parties to remain. There are other positions they might fill more acceptably. Kitchens, from which most of them came, call loudly for their return to more suitable employment. It does give them though a certain sort of standing among themselves. And I assure you they are quite an exclusive set among themselves, drawing the line severely against other outside employees often more worthy and always more refined since they have the advantage of associating with ladies even if it be in the capacity of servants. They have a dangerous power, too, and use it without stint when they can

do so without danger of being reported.

Oh, they are a vastly superior party of young ladies I assure you, and I once heard one of them, considered for several years one of the most trusty attendants in the house, say to a lady after having compelled her to wash half a dozen pairs of stockings for her, "You don't dare to put on any of your airs with me. I'm boss here (a favorite expression among the fraternity), and the State pays me eighteen dollars a month for making just such high-toned ladies as you wash for me!"

To their credit, be it said, there are honorable exceptions among them, and I was fortunate enough to be under the care of two most excellent girls, and I recall many acts of kindness that I bear in grateful remembrance. And it were well for attendants and others to bear in mind that kindness pays even among the insane. I remember every single kind word or act from the beginning, and I remember and resent yet, bitterly, every single cruelty.

One circumstance bearing upon this point I will relate. Both of my usual attendants were to be absent upon a certain occasion until midnight, and a detail from another ward was appointed to take charge of us. At that time and for some months previous I had been wearing restraints at night to prevent a repetition of an attempt to hang myself. The restraints consisted of leather wristlets through which was passed a belt crossing the hands and buckling around the waist.

Before Miss P. [the nurse] left the ward, she came to me and said, "Now, Mrs. Agnew, I want you to promise me you won't give anybody any trouble about your restraints tonight. Let them be put on quietly." And I promised I would. This matter of putting me upon my honor as to my promise always prevailed even in my craziest moments, but unfortunately few cared to treat me so respectfully. When these restraints were considered necessary in order that my valuable (?) life be saved, Dr. Hester ordered that they be arranged as comfortable as consistent with safety, and the girls were particular to observe his directions.

When bedtime came the detail [of attendants] put all the other patients to bed and left the ward for a short time returning with four great, strong girls from the back wards, and they came into my room, a mighty mutual protection squad, to assist in restraining a dangerous patient! and in spite of my tearful protestations that no force was necessary threw me upon the bed and drew my strap so tightly as almost to stop my breathing, and the wristlets almost cut into my arms; and they left me in that condition until Miss P. returned, at midnight.

As she was passing my door I called her and quickly relieving me she said as she looked at my poor swollen hands, "What damned fool did this?" And I said, "Oh, there were five of them. It took that many to protect themselves against one helpless woman." I never heard Miss P. swear before that time, but I'm sure I didn't think her any less the lady for swearing on that occasion.

Anna Agnew gave a balanced appraisal of hospital staff, complimenting some and expressing outrage toward others. Disturbed patients were more difficult to manage before modern medications became available to alleviate their symptoms. Anna Agnew described abusive attendants as seeing harsh measures as the only way to manage severely ill patients. The plea that an insane patient would respond appropriately to kindly treatment rather than to abuse was common in nineteenth-century asylum reform literature.

Although perception of class differences in the late nineteenth century was not necessarily the same as in the twentieth century, social standing was an important issue for Anna Agnew and her attendants. She was white, Protestant, the daughter of a family of business and professional people, the wife of a clerical worker, and thus part of a society that emphasized separate realms for men and women. Men left the home to work, as did her husband, and women functioned solely in the home, as she had done. Immigrant women

and and those from families of laborers were much more likely to
be employed in factories, domestic service, or jobs like hospital attendant. The power exercised by ward staff over patients, when
cruelly administered, probably represented in part their resentment
of their own difficult and poorly paid work in contrast to the apparent domestic comforts of those patients who seemed to be "putting
on airs."

Anna Agnew proposed specific reforms:

In every asylum in the land some such scenes are daily enacted,
and it will be so, must be, until state laws are so amended as to make
such abuses impossible. The willing hands and sympathetic hearts
of our noble band of superintendents and their corps of assistant
physicians must be encouraged and strengthened by furnishing them
experienced nurses in place of present thoughtless, heartless girls.
The establishment of suitable training schools will necessarily require time, but in the meantime there are hundreds of worthy needy
women, widowed mothers, who, having themselves suffered sorrow,
have pitying hearts toward their afflicted sisters.

Elsewhere she noted that she would: "speak freely of gross abuses,
for which there is no remedy, until state laws require that none but
those who are fitted for the sacred duties of attendants upon the
insane be employed—such preparation being a complete course in
a training school for nurses."
The commissioners of the hospital had noted in the 1878 annual
report: "As a condition of service in the Institution, we have required
of the employees fitness and faithful performance of duty—nothing more. It has been quite hard enough to get these, without adding another requisite to our standard of qualifications. Consequently,
during our official control, no one has been employed or dismissed

because of his or her political or religious convictions." They emphasized the importance in attendants of moral character, patience, gentleness, and like qualities.

The following year the trustees reported:

> *The Board is satisfied that the experience of the Association of American Superintendents as expressed in a resolution reiterated annually for many years, to the effect that some form of mechanical restraint is absolutely necessary to the well-being of the patients in some cases, is worthy of recognition, and it is further satisfied that restraint has been humanely applied in this institution, not excessively, and with a view solely to the good of the patient.*

The statue of Phillipe Pinel (1745-1826) at the Salpêtrière, Paris, depicts him surrounded by "insane" patients whom he had freed from their chains.

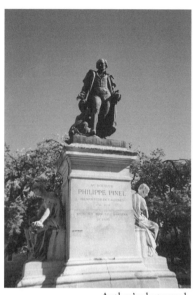

Author's photograph

Anna Agnew described the crib restraint.

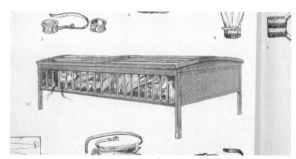

Indiana Medical History Museum

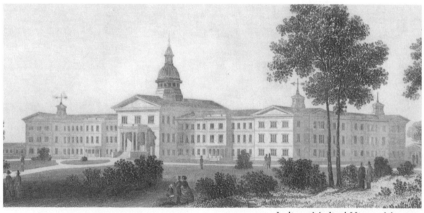

Indiana Medical History Museum

Thomas Kirkbride's book on asylums included an engraving of the Pennsylvania Hospital for the Insane at the time that he was superintendent in the nineteenth century.

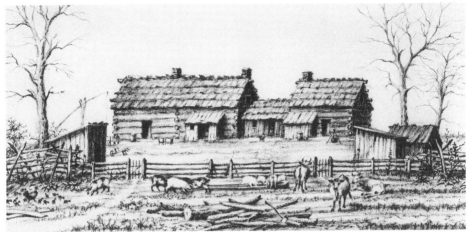

Early settlers' cabins near the center of Indianapolis were used as the first "crazy house" in the late 1820s.

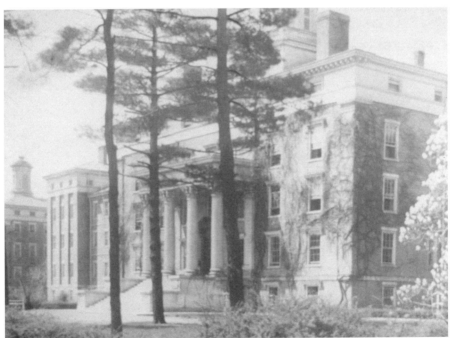

The first building of Indiana Hospital for the Insane was built in the late 1840s. It was called the Men's Building after the Women's Building was built in the late 1870s.

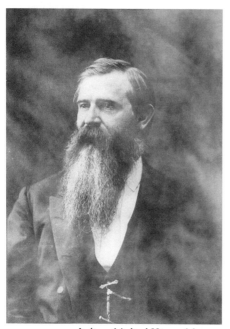

Dr. Orpheus Everts(1829-1903) was a "gentle-man of superior attainments" who said to Anna Agnew, "surely you will come from under the cloud."

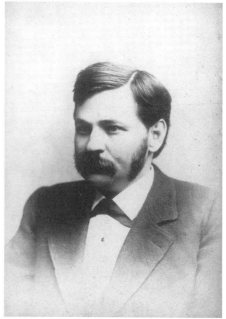

Dr. Joseph Goodwin Rogers (1841-1908) wrote to Anna Agnew, ". . . among . . . my former patients I know of none so endowed . . . with the ability to tell the story . . . ."

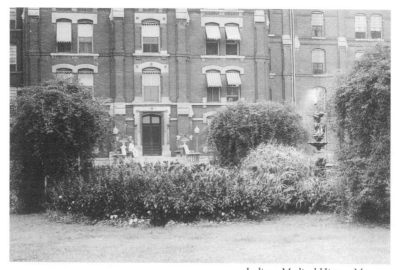

A later photograph of the front entrance of the Women's Building where Anna Agnew spent many of her years at Indiana Hospital for the Insane shows statuary and gardens that provided a "beneficial influence" on patients.

CHAPTER TWO

W͡ho was Anna Agnew?

Anna Keyt Agnew, born in 1836, was the second of Nathan and Martha Keyt's children. Her older brother, Frank, was a lawyer who died in his late twenties. A younger brother, William, was a steamboat clerk. He was living with his second wife across the Ohio River from Moscow, Ohio, in Covington, Kentucky, when Anna was in the hospital. Her sister Mary, whose husband Eugene Moore was a physician, died in 1883 as Anna perceived in a dream while in the hospital:

> Poor Mary! I have dreamed so often of her and of Eugene. I never think of them separately, and if I could but fix the date, I believe I had a dream that was a premonition of her death. It was about the middle of September [1883] the month she died, I thought I was standing watching them transplanting a large plant of Cape Jessamine, [sic] covered with its lovely creamy bloom; and as she stooped to lift it [she] said, "Oh, this horrible pain!" and sunk down at my feet. I awakened with her voice yet sounding in my ears, and I believe just at that moment she was dying. Oh! I hope some kind hand put white flowers in her coffin, and upon it, for few ever went to their grave in Moscow without flowers, which she so loved and carefully tended from her generous hand. And how her life was saddened by the one shadow amidst the fitful sunshine around her own hearthstone. She believed in prayer. I can see her now and hear her voice, as she supplicated, almost in agony, when she little thought

any eye was upon her, save his alone to whom she prayed, first for her own loved ones, and that the shadow might be removed from me, her afflicted sister.

Her youngest, favorite sister, Eliza ("Lida"), corresponded with Anna in the hospital and sent her gifts including some attractive clothing. She and her husband George Irwin visited Anna in the hospital. Living in Pittsburgh, they had been the only family not to see Anna during the years just before her hospitalization.

Anna Agnew described Moscow when she was growing up as a pleasant little town, situated on the bank of the beautiful Ohio River, thirty miles from Cincinnati. There were about eight hundred inhabitants, three stores [one of them her father's store], one blacksmith shop, one church [Methodist], and a seminary, and "the people were generally sober, and well behaved." After the original log building and a later brick building had been used as a school, the Moscow Seminary was established in 1845 [when Anna was eight or nine] by Francis Hamlin of Maine.

Before the Keyt children had married they had lived at home in Moscow with their parents, as was the custom of the time. Anna was an embroiderer and Mary, a seamstress, both suitable occupations for middle-class single women working in the home. Lida was for a time, before her marriage, a teacher. Although she was the eldest, Anna married later than her two younger sisters. She and David Agnew married in 1870, two years after the death of Anna's father Nathan Keyt at age seventy.

She might well have stayed in the home to care for an aging father. In a study of middle-class Midwestern families, social historian K. A. Tinsley found that before 1870, unmarried daughters were expected to remain in the parental home and when necessary care for aging parents. They were not expected to become self-supporting. Unmarried children often bore a disproportionate share of the burden of supporting elderly parents. Anna's close relationship with her father might also have contributed to her remaining at home and not marrying until her mid-thirties, after his death. Her mother, Nathan Keyt's second wife, was much younger than Nathan and apparently had a very different relationship with Anna than did her father, possibly adding to Anna's incentive to marry and leave home after her father's death.

In the book Anna Keyt Agnew wrote little of her mother, although she mentioned her father a number of times. At one point she noted:

> I was a proud, willful, and not always an obedient child. But to my father never intentionally disobedient or disrespectful. And from him I inherited my most pronounced traits of character, hence my inclination to confide in him more that in any other person. And I do not remember that if I ever went to him for sympathy that he did not try to lighten my burden (often an imaginary one, I must admit), instead of, on the contrary, reminding me that it was "my own fault, my own ugly temper," and so on_phrases grown so familiar from frequent repetition as to be heard and treated with contempt. It was not my own fault! It is no child's fault that it is cursed with an unhappy disposition. What greater misfortune could befall a child?"

Apparently her mother thought Anna had an ugly temper, suggesting an unhappy relationship developing between them early on and also suggesting some early symptoms of Anna's mood disorder that was to become more prominent later. Martha Eskham Keyt was only nineteen when Anna was born. The first of Martha's children had been born when she was seventeen and the last of six, before she was thirty. Tragically, but not unusual at the time, one of the children died young. Burdened with the busy duties of a young mother and the onerous tasks of housekeeping long before modern appliances, Martha Keyt had little time to bestow on individual children, especially the daughter who was "proud, willful, and not always obedient." No one at the time would have realized that this child was already suffering abnormal and troubling mood swings. Anna probably did not reveal her frightening nightmares.

In a letter to one of her sisters from the hospital, Anna wrote, "Tell mother, if she is still living, that it was ignorance of myself and not willful wickedness that made [me] give her more trouble than all the rest of her children." Her mother did not visit her in the hospital although other members of the family did.

When mentioning her visit to Moscow after hospitalization both in the book and in a letter to an Indianapolis newspaper, Anna wrote nothing specific about her mother who still lived there. The lack of closeness between mother and daughter might well have contributed to Anna's own very different style of mothering: "my children were my idols—I almost worshiped them." Losing them was all the more poignant and painful for Anna Agnew.

In all likelihood it was Nathan Keyt who encouraged his eldest daughter's interest in books, perhaps even taking her to Cincinnati to purchase the latest novels from the eastern United States and Europe. Anna Agnew received a common school (elementary) education at the seminary in Moscow, but her literary references in the book suggest that she was rather widely read, particularly in well-known literature. She included quotations from the Bible and such authors as John Bunyan, William Shakespeare, Alfred Lord Tennyson, Alexander Pope, Victor Hugo, Elizabeth Barrett Browning, Robert Burns, and Oliver Wendell Holmes. The quotations, most of which she would have found in the *McGuffey Sixth Reader*, suggest that she was especially fond of poetry.

After their marriages Anna's two sisters and their husbands had moved to Pittsburgh. Eugene Moore, who had been a physician in Clermont County, Ohio, practiced medicine in Pittsburgh only a couple of years before his wife died. He returned to Clermont County, Ohio, where his mother lived, and practiced medicine there until his death. Mary Keyt Moore is buried in the Moscow Cemetery, "the quiet graveyard on the hill," as are her brother Frank and their parents, Nathan and Martha Keyt.

David Agnew had moved to Cincinnati after his service in the Civil War. Anna mentioned their courtship in a letter years later:

> I once accompanied one whom I shortly after married to witness Joe Jefferson's delineation of the great good-for-nothing, drunken "Rip" [Van Winkle] with his everlasting 'That don't count,' and I think I expressed my sentiments in this regard [not weeping at plays] to my escort, and received this reply:
>
> "There is one scene in the play we will witness tonight that I shall not like you to see without a moistened eye." Well, I caught my breath a little over that, for I naturally wished just then to stand well in the estimation of the gentleman (?) I expected soon to be married to, and that was a real pretty, sensitive sort of sounding speech for him to make, considering our relation; so I prepared myself to be impressed_but oh, the perversity of my woman's heart! From the rising until the falling of the curtain, my sympathies were with poor, loving, high-tempered, greatly tried 'Gretchen,' and when that touching scene arrived that was to list my womanly sensibility, that was to dissolve me in ready tears, and that moistened the true (?) blue eyes beside me, when the outraged wife threw open the door and hurried out into the stormy darkness her drunken husband, my whole soul went out to her in sympathy, and I wanted to give her an encouraging pat on the shoulder and whisper in her ear: 'Don't you fret, Gretchen. A good wetting will sober him, and a good sleep will restore his senses, if he has any.' And so it proved. After his twenty years nap he did develop into quite a respectable sort of man, and in his later years recognized the pure gold in the character of Gretchen, his wife, and I guess they had a real comfortable old age together, after all.
>
> Since then tears are no strangers to my eyes, nor grief to my heart, and that man, after five years of marriage and after three little ones

called us parents, turned his back upon me in my extremity. That tender hearted one, so easily touched by the sorrows of a drunken husband, proved his claim to manhood, by being the one single exception in the rejoicing over the return of his wife from worse than the cruelty of the grave.

As Anna and David were courting in Cincinnati, the Middle West, now industrializing, was no longer a frontier. Anna's father's business as a merchant and her brother's employment as a steamboat clerk depended on the busy Ohio River traffic at midcentury. The Civil War and industrial development, however, brought railroads to prominence. It was with these that David and their three sons would find opportunity for employment and advancement.

Anna and David Agnew lived in Cincinnati after their marriage in 1870. Anna later described in a letter some of the difficulties of a newlywed:

I lived a year once in Cincinnati—went there from the country, away from the luxury of a wood cooking stove. And even now I shudder at the recollection of my first month's experience with coal. Oh, those dish cloths! Black and greasy and sticky—and my hands! Well, after years they recovered their normal condition and gradually I learned to manage my stove so that my kitchen looked quite as well as my neighbor's.

Anna and David Agnew's first son, named for Anna's father, was born in November 1872 in Ohio. In 1873, David and Anna moved to Seymour, Indiana, which was important as a railroad junction connecting four of the largest western cities. The east-west Ohio and Mississippi Railroad connecting Cincinnati and St. Louis crossed the north-south Jeffersonville, Madison, and Indianapolis Railroad running between Indianapolis and Louisville.

The Agnew's second son, William, was born in Seymour in 1873.

The family lived across from St. Ambrose Catholic Church. Father Anthony Schenck, a German priest, had just arrived there. The Agnew's little boy called him "Fadda Yank." The Sisters of Providence, one of whom later ministered to Anna in the hospital, operated the school associated with the church and later bought the house the Agnews had rented.

David and Anna's youngest son, David, was born in 1875 about the time that the family moved from Seymour to Vincennes, Indiana. Here the Ohio and Mississippi Railroad crossed the north-south Evansville and Terre Haute Railroad, one of several lines serially connecting Chicago and the South. The Ohio and Mississippi had large shops in Vincennes where David was first a timekeeper and later a clerk.

When David moved to Cincinnati after the divorce, the youngest son, David F. Agnew, was a student. At age fifteen he became a mechanic's helper. Later in his teens he was a clerk in the claims agent's office of the Ohio and Mississippi Railroad in Cincinnati in the 1890s.

The middle son, William, was a clerk at the Proctor and Gamble Company in Cincinnati but moved to Louisville, Kentucky, in 1895. There he was a clerk for the Baltimore and Ohio Southwestern Railroad, before moving to New Jersey. In the early twentieth century he lived less than thirty miles from the area of New Jersey that his great-grandfather John Keyt had left in the late eighteenth century.

The eldest son, Nathan Keyt Agnew, worked as a clerk in the auditor's office of the Ohio and Mississippi Railroad where his father David was chief clerk at the time. In 1895 he moved to Evansville, Indiana. He did very well in Evansville, becoming city passenger and ticket agent for the Evansville and Terre Haute Railroad, being elected an officer of a local chapter of the masons, and marrying a socially prominent young woman in 1901. Anna Agnew would have been delighted to attend the wedding as mother of the groom; another joy denied her by illness and social custom.

CHAPTER THREE

$\mathcal{M}$ood Swings

In ending her 1886 book *From under the Cloud* Anna Agnew wrote:

> I have written these reminiscences of my peculiarly saddened life from different motives; partly that it is a comfort and relief thus to give expression to my thoughts; partly hoping for pecuniary assistance; but my purest, best motive is the sincere hope of raising the drooping, hopeless spirit and strengthening the fainting heart of some other miserable victim of this fearful horror, insanity; since certainly none should despair of recovery in view of my coming out "From Under the Cloud."

Anna Agnew described in her own experience most of the symptoms now included in the official, researched-based diagnosis of bipolar disorder that includes episodes of both depression and mania. (Major depressive disorder includes episodes of depression, only.) Mood disorders are described in the *Diagnostic and Statistical Manual of Mental Disorders, Fourth Edition, Text Revision*, of the American Psychiatric Association:

Depressive Episodes involve five or more of the following symptoms lasting at least two weeks and representing a change from previous functioning: Depressed mood most of the day; Markedly diminished pleasure or interest in almost all activities; changes in appetite and/or weight (char-

acteristically poor appetite and often severe weight loss but in other cases overeating and weight gain without real enjoyment of food); Changes in sleep patterns: insomnia (decreased sleep) or hypersomnia (increased sleep) nearly nightly; changes in the speed of moving and thinking: slowing (psychomotor retardation) or increased rapidity of speech and movement (psychomotor agitation) that is observable by others; fatigue or loss of energy almost daily; feelings of worthlessness or excessive guilt; difficulty concentrating and making decisions; thoughts of death or plans and attempts at suicide. (Up to12 to 15 percent, if untreated, eventually die by their own hands).

Manic Episodes *involve abnormally and persistently elevated mood and three or more of the following symptoms: Inflated self-esteem or grandisoity; decreased need for sleep, not just insomnia or poor sleep (depressed patients suffer from inability to sleep; manic patients usually enjoy being awake and active most of the night); more talkative than usual or the experience of pressure to keep talking; racing thoughts or "flight of ideas" (rapidly straying away from the initial topic although some connection is apparent from topic to topic); distractibility (attention is readily focused on every little occurrence in the environment); increased activity or hyperactivity (social, work related, or sexual); excessive involvement in pleasurable activities that have a high potential for painful consequences (e.g. buying sprees, sexual indiscretions, foolish business ventures, etc.).*

Pediatric psychiatrists now recognize that mood disorders can begin in childhood. Anna Agnew experienced days of abnormal moods in childhood but no one at the time recognized her condition:

And I can recall days of gloom—when too young yet to have even heard of the traditional silver lined clouds—the memory of which even now makes me shudder that a child should be so hopeless even for one moment! . . .. To escape if possible from the terrible shadowy something constantly haunting me, whose influence made itself felt in my happiest moments giving character even to my dreams, and whose climax was insanity! I often wonder now if my life might not have been different—surely it would have brighter—had there been some one to whom I could have unbosomed myself . . ..

My readers must not infer from the preceding that I was an altogether unhappy girl; for indeed such was far from being the fact. Few persons, I think, possessed a keener sense of enjoyment or had brighter hours than I, only they were not uniformly so—and unusual gayety [sic] was too frequently followed by melancholy.

She described the first several years of her marriage as being happy, apparently symptom free. Then she began to experience ever more frequent and severe depressions:

On the night of November-nineteenth-seventy six, I sat sewing upon a garment for one of my children until quite late but put it away not quite done! And I never finished it! Something had come over me! I wakened the following Sunday morning bathed in a cold, clammy perspiration with an inexpressibly horrible sensation as though falling-falling into some dreadful place of darkness! I had not the strength to speak or move! And a cold shadowy something seemed settling down upon me—indescribable but altogether horrible!

When fully awake I recognized my condition! For the second time within the year I was completely helpless from nervous prostration! And, startling as a flash of lightning in a clear sky, came the revelation, this something that had been with me all my life walking by my side, invisible but felt even in my happiest moments, haunting me and threatening to overwhelm me at some unexpected happy moment had come, and it was insanity!

And then it was as has so heartlessly been said of me, "I deliberately folded my hands and announced my intention of being sick." My hands were folded, my work taken out of them. But it was not I did it. They were busy helping hands before. A power stronger than mine made them helpless. They were horribly folded and for six miserable years only busied themselves in fruitless attempts to end my wretched existence. All life, all beauty, all brightness was gone from me! And yet I could not die . . ..

As I prepared myself for church . . . every breath was a prayer for help or comfort. But no comfort came! The sermon and walk home seemed a confused and troubled dream. Until just as we reached home, my little son whom I had taken with me, stepped forward to open the gate and said, "Mamma, aren't you glad to have a big boy like me to take you to church when papa's not at home?" And I said, "No, Dadie, mamma don't feel as though she could ever be glad again—of anything." Dear little fellow! He was only six years old . . .. Little child as he was, he felt the difference in my manner.

There could be no better description of the onset, in this case sudden, of an episode of major depression. Both Anna Agnew and her son recognized a change from previous functioning. She noted that it would last for years. Her mood was certainly depressed. Although she was very fond of her children, she had no interest in them, even in her son. Psychomotor retardation prevented her from doing anything. She was unable to concentrate; she felt confused even walking home from church. She felt extreme fatigue, no strength to speak or move. Sitting up late at night might well have been a result of the insomnia.

Episodes of mood disorders might begin suddenly, as this one did, or gradually. They might last days, weeks, months, or years if untreated. Anna Agnew had had days of abnormal mood in childhood. She had experienced a briefer episode in the year prior to this episode. The current episode would last years into her hospitalization.

Later in the book she described her continuing depression in the early years of her hospitalization:

How gladly I would pass silently over the incidents of the three following years. I hesitate to put upon record the events of these years of mental darkness, degradation and despair. Even now my nights are rendered sleepless at the review of them. When by the resurrecting eye of memory these ghosts of my sad past go flitting by, I shiver and grow cold at the recollection of the depths into which I was driven. Even self-respect, that last hope of womanhood, almost extinguished—every single sin of the [Ten Commandments] was involuntarily assumed, and I felt the consequent condemnation more keenly, I presume, than would have been the case had I in reality been guilty of their violation. I had been an inmate of the asylum about nine months and was standing one morning as I frequently did at the window, wishing oh so anxiously, for a newspaper . . . my special craving for the daily news was to gratify a morbid curiosity that I had to know how far my infernal influence extended, which influence, I believed to be the direct cause of the numerous murders, suicides, and various other outrages, together with all sorts of calamities of land and water, mind and nerve, not excepting the occasional earthquake.

Her guilt had reached a delusional stage. Most episodes of mood swings are not psychotic, but this one clearly was. Psychosis is characterized by delusions, false beliefs that are firmly sustained despite obvious evidence to the contrary, and hallucinations, sensory perceptions that seem very real but occur without external stimulation. Elsewhere she described loss of appetite that reached the point of hallucinations about her food: "the moment I was seated at the table, every single article would become alive, creeping, squirming vermin of all disgusting characters was in the food put upon my plate. . . . I could not put those vile things into my mouth."

She wrote in another part of the book of her severe self-depreciation even though she was aware that other patients did not share her negative delusions about herself:

I believe the patients generally liked me, at any rate I was made the recipient of many a tale of woe and petitioned for sympathy at the same time feeling myself the whole cause of all the misery surrounding me. Call this morbid nonsense, pretentious ignorance if you please; to me it was painfully real, and I used to wonder why those poor wretches did not realize what I was, did not recognize my fearful influence and rid the world of such a monster by tearing me limb from limb. So deeply did I feel that I was set apart as the "evil one" that I felt compelled to write to my sister to this effect, and in the letter shown me after my recovery I read this terrible renunciation: "I have no mother, brothers, sisters, husband, nor children! I must stand alone, now and forever! And as my pen leaves that word forever, I claim it as mine. No one else has a right to use it. It is mine since I of all humanity understand its complete meaning, its fearful significance! The struggle is between the Almighty and myself and will last forever! I am under the horrid wheel, almost crushed! Not quite! The Hand has me in its powerful grasp, but I can still struggle, and I WILL!"

The wheel and the Hand had reference to a tormenting repeated dream that in my childhood haunted me, making my nights fearful. Let me try and recall this dream. In the distance would appear a wheel not larger than a silver dollar which, revolving rapidly, growing larger at each revolution until its dimensions were monstrous when it reached me, would seem about to crush me to atoms, but just at this point some power would stop it, and it would grind and grind with a horrible noise, as tho' angry that its vengeance was stayed, and slowly it would roll backward. Again, a hand seemingly not larger than an infant's would appear in the space above, growing larger and fearfully strong as it approached with outstretched fingers as tho' to clutch me, poor frightened child, by the throat, and I would awaken shivering with fear and would pray that such terrible things be not sent me.

I had a child's faith then, and believed that which we prayed for would be granted unto us because He said so! This determined I *will*! And I will *not* adhered to through the succeeding years of torture, mental and physical; this unbending resolution *not* to be trampled into the dirt even though I be in the deepest slough of insanity; the stinging sense of the injustice of the undeserved contempt with which I was treated made me solemnly swear that sometime I would make my persecutors feel the strength of the womanhood within me however deeply it was then sunken!

In the hospital she also had an episode of mania characterized by a delusion about the Masons:

> I had a so-called "period of excitement"—that of raving insanity. I was conscious of my inability to control myself! Knew I was screaming, laughing and praying without the power to stop. And through it all right into my poor dazed brain rang this sentence, constantly repeated in a horribly mocking tone: "By every art known to scientific druggists shall thy body be tortured and thy soul tormented by a secret known only to the Jews." From whence came this warning—for warning it certainly was. I can not answer but I do know that promises of threatened torment and consequent torture followed speedily. The "secret" I yet believe meant masonry. And during the remaining years of my insanity some of my most pronounced and peculiar delusions were connected with that order of which my father was for many years an honored member and at that time I was a mason's wife!

Delusions obviously include bizarre notions but are related to real experiences in a delusional patient's life. Anna Agnew's father and husband were Masons. Her mania included excitement and laughing, pressure to keep screaming and praying that she could not resist, and the feeling that she was out of control.

She described the lifting of a depression that represented a swing into mania, noting that even a "refined, delicately brought-up" woman would use profane expletives:

And what an exquisite relief it is to pent-up feeling! What a safety valve to boiling rage at one's self and all the world so miserably unconscious of the victim's mental torture! I know when the time came after years of self debasement, self condemnation, when I could not so much as lift a finger or an indignant glance to show my deep resentment of outraged feeling! When the time came when I could turn upon my tormentors, friends or foes, with a threatening jesture [sic] and an emphatic "Go to hell! God damn you!"

Certainly had her enjoyment of swearing and threatening even friends occurred outside the hospital it would have represented involvement in activities that have a high potential for painful consequences, a symptom of mania.

At another point she described:

Feelings of intense excitement of which I was compelled to give utterance of some sort. If there was a chair or any thing within my reach that I could break, or failing in that, a window through which I could dash my hand, and if blood came all the better, the paroxysm would soon pass over. Heretofore, such relief had been obtained by swearing, horribly swearing too though sometimes inaudibly.

Suicide and Homicide

Anna Agnew described the events leading up to her hospitalization:

After already having, at different times, [before hospitalization] swallowed an ounce of laudanum, four ounces of a preparation of chloral the regular dose of which was one teaspoonful, a tablespoonful of pulverized sugar of lead which latter thoroughly poisoned me until my tongue, throat and stomach were in ulcers—I repeat, after having swallowed all these, I threw myself upon the mercy of two prominent physicians [in her hometown] who were called in consultation upon my case, telling them I was all the time tempted to kill myself and was afraid I might hurt some one else, and I begged for their advice. In return for my sincere confidence, this brutal remark was made: "You might put a quart of poison on that mantelpiece with perfect safety. Persons who are contemplating suicide don't advertise the fact."

Some months later these same gentlemen (?) were called to attend me after I had swallowed strychnine in sufficient quantity to "kill an elephant, if properly administered," as the druggist from whom I bought it said when he sold it to me for the purpose of killing rats. One of these physicians, "the head" saw me at the beginning of the case when every nerve was convulsively twitching and with the remark that it was perfectly wonderful what had gotten me into such a nervous state. But he rather guessed it was hysteria, gave me a dose of bromide of potassium and left quite a quantity to be given.

It is a frightening misunderstanding to assume that people who intend to commit suicide never mention it. Most do. Anna Agnew was not kidding. Up to fifteen percent of patients with major depressive episodes, if untreated, take their own lives. Leaving a large amount of medicine with a potentially suicidal patient is not currently considered the best of medical practice.

Strychnine, a stimulant, was used in medicines at the time. In large doses it causes convulsions. Bromide salts were among the few anticonvulsants available at the time. It is not clear whether potassium bromide was given to alleviate her very real convulsions or as a sedative for her "hysteria." Her family physicians followed the practice of the day of attributing psychiatric symptoms in women to their naturally nervous temperaments. The physicians' attitudes might well have contributed to her husband's idea that her suicidal behavior was feigned.

> I am branded upon the hospital records with a name worse than that of murderess! It is shameful and cruel in the extreme that I am recorded "homicidal."
>
> Suicidal I *was*, in thought and intention, for years! But no thought of *murder* was in my heart when attempting the deed that consigned me to the asylum for the insane. On the contrary, it was an effort to save my child from the fearful (possible) heritage of insanity! And my desperation was intensified by cruel insinuation and vile, abusive taunts from those surrounding me whose public professions were of sympathy, but whose private acts were those of fiends! I reasoned thus (for insane persons *do* reason, sometimes fearfully to the point, too): That it were far better that I lay all my little ones at rest than that they live to become victims of a fate than which death is a positive, welcome guest. That was my horror then! But I do not fear that fate for them now.

Although readily admitting to serious suicide attempts, Anna Agnew maintained throughout the book that she had never been homicidal. Severely depressed parents, however, do sometimes take their children's lives before committing suicide in the mistaken belief that they have ruined everything for the children, and she had been reported to have given one of the children laudanum. As would be expected, Anna Agnew no longer had the delusion of having ruined things for her children when she had recovered from depression. The charge of homicide, however, would have ominous implications for her and her three sons.

Illness and Marriage
When she described the depression that led to her hospitaliza-

tion, Anna Agnew sounded a mordant opening note in a dissonant theme that was to be played out in her marriage. The statement in her book, "I deliberately folded my hands and announced my intention of being sick," clearly referred to her husband's belief that she was feigning illness.

Untreated psychiatric illness can take a terrible toll on a marriage. Anna, having suffered mood swings she did not understand as a child, now saw that they were early signs of what would become insanity in her adult life. Over the years her symptoms worsened and became unbearable. She feared that her beloved children would meet the same fate.

Her husband realized that his wife was becoming more and more insane and now seemed to be trying to harm the children. The hostilities had begun but, like Anna Agnew's illness, they would fluctuate. Anna Agnew's husband, by her account, never understood what she was experiencing. One of the local doctors said that she should be sent to the penitentiary although he signed papers for her commitment to the Indiana Hospital for the Insane. His professional advice that her husband should enter criminal prosecution against her would not have helped her husband's understanding of the situation.

She described many facets of her relationship with her husband:

When I was married, I sincerely loved my husband! And my children were my idols—I almost worshiped them. And until this trouble came, I was happier, more contented than in all my previous life. I must say *trouble*, yet it was not domestic trouble. I do not now, and never have, held my husband responsible for my affliction in any intentional manner. The domestic trouble phase was of recent date. I am glad to have the memory of a pleasant, comfortable, peaceful home—the few years I was permitted to enjoy it. And, when comparing, as I am obliged truthfully to do, my husband as he was then (thoughtful and careful of my comfort ever) with the

Anna Agnew's Husband

Born in 1843 in Philadelphia, David Agnew was five and one-half feet tall and of delicate frame. His parents, probably laborers or farmers, were relative latecomers among the Scotch Irish in Philadelphia, having left Ireland early in the nineteenth century. They were proud to identify with the heritage of the family name that had been traced by some back to William the Conqueror. Anna Agnew referred in her book to the "old Irish Presbyterian family of which I became a member by marriage." Like Anna Agnew's grandfather John Keyt before them, Agnews moved west to Ohio. David Agnew was a clerk in Carrollton, Ohio, in his late teens.

He spent the years from age nineteen to twenty-one in the 98th Ohio Infantry of the Union army in the Civil War. No doubt he was all too familiar with the perception at the time that those seeking removal from the front lines on the basis of psychological difficulties were all malingerers. Soldiers who appeared to be in a deranged state were referred to as "shirkers." War experience no doubt played a part in his later harsh treatment of an insane wife whose illness he could not comprehend.

The 98th Ohio Infantry was formed at Camp Steubenville, Ohio, in August 1862 and pursued Confederate General Braxton Bragg across Kentucky. After the battle of Perryville on October 8 it moved to duty in Lebanon, Kentucky, until December. It chased the infamous Confederate raider John Hunt Morgan through Kentucky in late December 1862 and early January 1863. Next, the regiment moved to Louisville as Union forces successfully regained command of the Ohio River region. Then the 98th went on to Franklin, Tennessee. It was in Franklin from February to June 1863 guarding Union occupied territory and participating in sporadic skirmishes.

David Agnew was in a military hospital in Franklin in March 1863 due to illness, probably one of the many infectious diseases that were untreatable in the Civil War era and that were ultimately responsible for half of the deaths in his division. He was then detailed as a clerk. One of his officers wrote, "David Agnew has always been a faithful soldier while with his Company. He is a young man of delicate frame, and scarcely able to endure the fatigue of active campaigning. Under these circumstances I would be glad to have him remain in his present position [as clerk]."

He served from July 1863 until his discharge in May 1865 as a clerk in the mustering officer's office in Nashville, Tennessee. A letter from his commanding officer to the Adjutant General's office of the Department of the Cumberland in January 1864 reported, "Corporal Agnew has been on duty with me since July 1863 and has proved efficient and faithful in a more than ordinary degree, and having been so long upon this duty is fully informed as to the manner and forms of transacting business in the mustering department now necessarily become intricate and complicated."

Some of David Agnew's later anger about his wife's illness might have been related to the fact that a "man of delicate frame" depended on the emotional support of a wife who was six years his senior. His conscientious attention to his work, carried over into civilian life, necessitated a strong woman in the home caring for their children. The incapacitation of this strong wife, to say nothing of her apparent threat to their children, might well have been almost as devastating for David as it was for Anna. His feelings seem to have been reflected in a punitive attitude towards Anna.

man who, only a few months since, refused me even the privilege of seeing our children and brutally bade me "go to the Knox county poor-house for support" rather than into his house and the society of our children, it is small wonder that I feel I have but recently formed his real acquaintance and the fact that for five years or more I thought my husband a gentleman must be sadly laid away among other kindred "delusions."

Unfortunately for all concerned, I was not taken to the asylum for a period of several years after the time when common sense, if not common humanity, should have decided that such was the only proper place for me. Right here let me implore those persons so unfortunate as to have friends needing such restraint not to cherish the old-timed ignorant idea of some thing disgraceful being attached to this form of affliction; and above all keep from the stricken one the shadow of reflection that they have disgraced their family since they are insane. The bitterest, most indignant feelings toward my friends were born of this very thought.

I sincerely believe that the miserable record of those years, the impressions made and received by me when my case was so cruelly, or ignorantly, which? misunderstood outside of the asylum, made seven years inside of its walls a necessity for which I must hold my immediate family in a measure responsible, granting at the same time they intended kindness to me in keeping me home. But I was neither treated as an insane, nor yet wholly responsible woman. Often, not with the consideration shown a willful child. At times charged with being a hypocrite. Of feigning insanity to evade the responsibilities of my home duties. Of acting the fool. . . .

. . . when I made the attempt at hanging myself in my room at the asylum, and Dr. Hester notified my husband, at the same time telling him to be prepared at any time to hear of my death, as I seemed to think of nothing else, he inclosed [sic] the doctor's letter to my sister adding, "As for me, I never did take any stock in that suicide theory, nor do I now"⁻(an opinion he still clings to, I believe). . .

The wilderness, into which I was driven by cruel Fate, aided and abetted by heartless brutality within my own immediate household, was the Asylum for the Insane. Bearing upon my body suggestive marks, silent witnesses of blows not given alone by the tongue, I envy not that person her peace of mind, if she possesses a conscience, who by her insulting taunts and vile insinuations continued and persisted in for three days before I, in my desperation, was driven to the act for which I am called an "homicide," a person, too, to whom I had never shown aught but kindness, to whom often I had extended generous hospitality when my home was a pleasant place to come to.

The only reference suggesting who the woman was that made "insulting taunts and vile insinuations" came near the end of the book and mentioned her husband's sister. During the final year of her hospitalization, which was apparently prolonged by the doctors so that she would not have to go to the county poor house as her husband suggested, Anna Agnew was employed in the sewing room for a small sum monthly. She reported that she:

Spent my first month's pay in some little articles for my children but was positively, and most peremptorily forbidden by my husband to send them since, using his own language, "I will not allow them to receive any thing from you, neither will I allow them to be reminded that you still live; let them forget your last days spent with them if they can! Let them forget if they can!"

And in reply I wrote, "Have you forgotten the three days previous to the last day spent with them and the entertainment gotten up by you, their father, for the benefit of your sister? A little seven year old boy knocked down by your fist and dragged screaming into an adjoining room, where, after the key was turned upon me, his insane mother, he was ordered to strip off his coat 'and get down upon his knees,' when he was whipped like a dog with a leather strap, I in the meantime being entertained by language such as I had not then thought could pass a woman's lips and which I still think unsurpassed in vileness by any insane raving heard since. What was his offense? Simply because that little child had, with his brother—still younger—gone downtown to see Barnum's circus come in instead of going (as good little Christians following in the footsteps of their pious paternal ancestors) to Sunday-school.

At one point Anna Agnew reported that her husband had written to her sister that she was an "opium eater." "A drug I never even so much as tasted, to my knowledge," Anna asserted. The only mention of opioid drugs in the book is in connection with her overdose of laudanum while severely depressed prior to admission and when morphine was prescribed by doctors in the hospital to alleviate pain.

She reported two visits by her husband to her during her years in the hospital. The first was while she was ruminating about her delusions of guilt that she had committed all sorts of terrible crimes:

Just at this moment our supervisoress touched my arm and said, "Come with me, Mrs. Agnew," and walking down the hall to my room, opened the door, and there stood my husband. I think, for a moment or so, I never was so happy. It was his first visit to me. And only a moment ago I was feeling so utterly wretched and alone. But now my husband had come, and he did care something for me after all. After I had entered the room and closed the door, he stood looking at me but not speaking a word until I said, "For heaven's sake, don't stand there staring at me in such a manner as that; sit down and say something to me; ask me something or I shall scream through sheer nervousness."

So he took the chair I offered him, drew it closely up to mine and gazing into my eyes said: "Were you insane when you were married?" Not one single little word of kindness or jesture [sic] of tenderness, not the shadow of a greeting; simply this cruel, calculating question. Evidently he had even then formed the determination that I should never leave that asylum alive. I did not then think this, however, and answered most assuredly, "I was not insane when we were married."

I have changed my opinion since then, materially, and willingly admit I was insane, and my most pronounced symptom was that I married him. After a time I said, "Have you nothing to say to me? Can't you tell me something of my children?" "Your children!" he replied. "Why, I hadn't an idea you cared to hear from them. You don't certainly presume to profess to love them?" Oh, it was inhuman to so torture a poor helpless woman; yet I doubt if in his egotism he realized my suffering. He asked if I wished to see my children, and I said, "No, I did not dare to see them," and this, I presume, was additional proof to his charitable (?) soul of my hatred of my children, and he said, "Very well; I will never bring those children to see you until you ask me to."

After obtaining permission from the physician in charge, he took me out walking and while there, my outraged feelings got the better of my pride, and I charged him with having lost all regard or affection for me, and he answered, "Oh, no, Anna, you are quite mistaken; I love you just as well as I ever did;" and then followed rapid questions to which he demanded answers that proved the nature of his regard for me, past and present, and from that moment my faith in his purity was a thing of the past. Another "delusion" gotten clear of.

Legal grounds for divorce in Indiana at the time were adultery, impotency at the time of marriage, abandonment for two years, cruelty, habitual drunkenness, failure of the husband to provide reasonable provision for the family for a period of two years, and conviction subsequent to marriage in any county of either party of an infamous crime. Her husband might well have been thinking about her giving medication to her child as an infamous crime although she had been committed to the hospital rather than being charged with a crime. Anna Agnew later charged him with desertion.

She described his last visit, December 17, 1883, and an argument they had, continuing:

> He spent a portion of the afternoon with me, and during the time I insisted that he should read a number of letters written me by my sister in which she urged me to keep up good heart, and I would soon be able to go home to my family. He said, "You seem from these replies to have written very freely to your sister." And as he was leaving he said: "I reckon you won't write to me!"
>
> One month later . . . finding myself greatly improved I wrote him quite a lengthy letter, wrote just as kindly as I felt. Told him how much better I was and how encouraged I felt at the prospect of getting well, and at the close asked him particularly to send me his and the children's pictures. Then, more because he had been very profuse in his offers to send me any thing I needed than that I positively needed the things, since the state furnished patients those necessaries, I asked him to send me a good pair of glasses and some postage stamps. This letter I did not keep a copy of. I was writing to my husband and did not consider it necessary. I am wiser since.
>
> Within three days his answer came. A scrap of blank paper, inclosing twenty-eight cents in postage stamps in a sealed envelope directed to me! I immediately returned him a note for the same amount of stamps payable to him or his order one day after date and within a month was out of his debt. And the battle had opened between us!

Many skirmishes had led up to this battle. There had been intermittent efforts at negotiation on both sides. Bipolar disorder, her husband's lack of understanding of it, and her difficulty in communicating how she really felt finally brought their relationship to the endgame: divorce.

Anna Agnew did have one visit with her children. Soon after her discharge from the hospital, she went to visit them in Aurora, Indiana, where they were living with their father:

> It matters not what the future hold for me, nothing can take from me the sweet memory of that meeting, when my three little boys rushed into my arms, with tears and smiles, struggling for the ascendance, repeating over and again, as though glad of the opportunity to use the dear name of mother, "Mamma, mamma, don't cry so, we are so glad to see you."
>
> Glad to see me· and was I not glad too, after seven years of cruel separation! [In] spite of bitter persecution—against all influence brought to bear upon those children to induce them to believe either they had no mother, or that she had willfully, wickedly forsaken them; had gotten tired of her home, of her family; had lost or had never possessed the instincts of wife or mother; "had deliberately planned this matter;" had willingly gone to the asylum, where for seven years she had "feigned insanity"—[in] spite of all this, when "mamma," strong in her love for her children, through her own determination, was granted permission to test her children's memory, she had her blessed reward. By persistent searching, repeated tests, she received assurance that through all her children remembered their mother as she was, before this trouble came and, too, that they would gladly have her back to stay with them always. But it was not to be. She dedicated the book:

This Volume is Affectionately Dedicated to MY CHILDREN·
My heart will still cling to them fondly,
And dream of sweet memories past;
While hope, like the rainbow of promise,
Gives assurance of meeting at last.

Divorce in Aurora

While Anna was in the hospital in 1883, David and the boys moved to Aurora, Indiana, near Cincinnati. Their arrival occurred soon after of one of the most severe of the frequent floods of the Ohio River struck the area. Rising water in February 1883 had damaged nearly half the houses in Aurora. Not long after their move, one of the boys fell from a tree and broke both his arms, adding to the turmoil of his young life and to David's concerns as a single parent. Anna did not mention the incident and might not have known of it. It was later in 1883 that David visited her in the hospital for the last time, and they had one of their increasingly hostile interactions.

The Ohio and Mississippi Railroad traveled through Aurora. As in Vincennes, David Agnew rented a house near the railroad depot. By this time he had been promoted to clerk in the auditor's office. Aurora is on a part of the Ohio River that offers a view of the earliest part of the sunrise, the aurora. In contrast, the prospects in Aurora for the Agnew's marriage and Anna's return to her sons were not bright.

Anna Agnew brought suit for divorce against David on the grounds of desertion and failure to provide. She had him arrested, August 17, 1885, under the criminal law for desertion and failure. She had chosen a prominent law firm in the area, McMullen and Roberts, to represent her. Both of her attorneys had served in the state legislature and had held prominent local offices. Hugh D. McMullen had been prosecuting attorney, and Omar F. Roberts had been a circuit court judge.

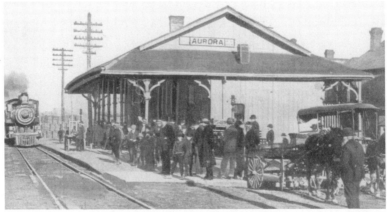

Picture from Alford's Antiques, Aurora, Ind., est. ca. 1890

Anna Agnew's first view of Aurora would have been of the depot of the Ohio and Mississippi Railroad for which David Agnew worked as a clerk in the auditor's office.

On September 3, 1885, the Aurora Spectator, reported "Six Divorce suits will engage the attention of the Dearborn Circuit Court during the session this month. A peculiar feature of all six is that all the plaintiffs are the wives, not a single husband appearing as plaintiff. The inference must follow that either the women are becoming more easily dissatisfied or the men are becoming more unbearable. In the complaints filed the husbands are charged with all manner of cussedness against their amiable and blameless wives." Feminists were not to become prominent for many decades. Their predecessors in the suffragist movement were still viewed by most in 1885 in the same light as the wives seeking divorce in Dearborn County. Anna, herself, seemed ambivalent about suffragists.

Divorce proceedings took place in September 1885 in the Greek revival courthouse in Lawrenceburg. Although Anna obtained a divorce from David, her efforts to have him prosecuted for desertion were unsuccessful in spite of her accomplished lawyers. Undoubtedly her long hospitalization and the charge of having been homicidal were unfavorable to her in any legal proceedings. Courts were only beginning to recognize rights of mothers for custody of their children after divorce and tended to favor mothers of children under seven years of age. David retained custody of the boys who were by then adolescents and had lived with their father and housekeepers for seven years. They had seen their mother only once since she had been admitted to the hospital when she had visited Aurora earlier in 1885 after her discharge from the hospital.

In trying to obtain custody of, or even a right to see her children, Anna was fighting both the laws of the time and ignorance about psychiatric illness that did not take into account the nature of her attempt to give medication to her son. Such behavior would no longer be present when her illness had remitted. Long before the divorce she had lost any propensity to act drastically to protect her children from potential insanity.

Soon after the divorce David and the boys moved to nearby Cincinnati, where he became chief clerk in the auditor's office of the Ohio and Mississippi Railroad. After working for the Ohio and Mississippi for nearly thirty years, David would experience the effects of corporate mergers at the turn of the century. In 1893 the O. and M. was sold to the Baltimore and Ohio Southwestern Railroad. David transferred from being chief clerk in the auditor's office of the O. and M. to a position as freight and ticket accountant for the B. and O. SW. The Baltimore and Ohio Railroad bought that line in 1900. From 1900 through 1909, David worked as a clerk in the freight office of the Cincinnati, Hamilton, and Dayton Railroad, which was later a part of the Baltimore and Ohio.

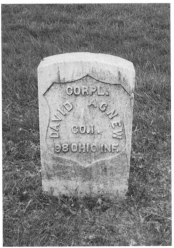

Author's photograph

David and Anna Agnew remained separated in death as in life. David Agnew died in December 1911 from pneumonia at the Soldiers' Home in Dayton, Ohio, and is buried among his comrades in the beautiful National Cemetery in Dayton.

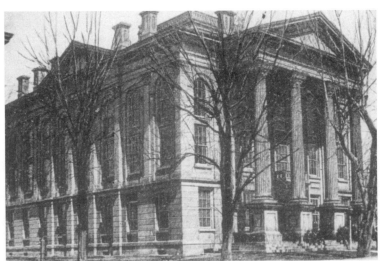

Picture from Alford's Antiques, Aurora, IN, est. ca. 1890

The Agnew's divorce proceedings took place in the Dearborn County Courthouse, Lawrenceburg, Indiana

CHAPTER FOUR

$\mathcal{N}$ ot So Moral Treatment

Villainess

Moral treatment was the accepted treatment in insane asylums in the nineteenth century in America, but many of the attendants who cared for Anna Agnew and others in similar institutions were uninformed of it or purposely chose to ignore it. A supervisor of attendants whom Anna Agnew referred to throughout the book only as "Madame C." showed no evidence of familiarity with moral treatment:

> There was a vacancy in the fourth ward, a very desirable position, too, since it was a front ward, nicely furnished, plenty of flowers, well drilled servants (wash-women included); a fine Steinway piano and a good class of patients excepting the devil [Anna Agnew when severely depressed]. The choice fell upon a woman upon one of the back wards, a married woman who frequently quoted "my husband" since the possession of such an appendage does give a sort of importance to a sort of woman even though he does not support her. I never saw that woman before she came on the ward shortly before supper-time. . . .
>
> All over the house she had the reputation of being such a sweet woman. Oh, she could play the piano so nicely, my! At night when unlocking the sleeping-rooms, as she came to mine she said to one of the patients sitting near, "Who sleeps here?" And upon being told

it was my room, she opened the door and deliberately spit a great nasty mess into my room. This was my introduction to Madame C., the pink of perfection. Do you wonder that I hated her from that moment. . . .

One day while in the dining-room at dinner I had occasion to leave the room and had only barely reached the [water]closet when the detail [of attendants] followed me and as usual ordered me to return to the dining-room. I was not in a condition to return and sat down on a chair saying I could not go back there, and she answered, "Go this moment, or I'll drag you there," and she seized me by the arm and as I fell dragged me full length lying on my back into the dining-room, the distance being the length of the short hall. Just as she had gotten me across the threshold Madame C. sprang up and said: "Don't let her go back to her place at the table; make her lie there so the 'ladies' (this was the term used to designate the patients, and I detest the sound of it) can walk over her when they are dismissed from the dining-room." And, "ladies," turning toward their tables, "every single one of you spit on her as you pass out."

Spitting seemed her strong weapon of insult, and in my fearful anger I attempted to spit on her, a vain attempt though; for in times of such angry excitement there is no saliva secreted¯the tongue becomes so parched and the throat so constricted that it is almost an impossibility to cry out. But the attempt was sufficient provocation. She sprang upon me as I lay upon the floor, calling at the same time for the detail to sit upon my lower limbs, and she pressed both hands with all her strength against my head almost flattening my face against the hard floor at the same time bearing the weight of her whole body directly upon my chest, one of her knees being planted squarely upon my left breast. When my agony became insupportable I cried, "Oh do have mercy; you are crushing my breast." And she answered: "It's a pity about your ____." And the name she used does not apply to a woman's breast.

But she got off me, and I struggled to my feet when they seized me again and began the usual torture of twisting my arms, and I can assure the uninitiated that it does not require more than two twists from brutal hands to bring the poor victims to their knees, a devotional attitude not usually under such circumstances attended with prayer, most frequently with oaths from the victim and vile, insulting expletives from the young ladies! While struggling with me, trying to make me promise I would "behave myself," something no one ever did succeed in making me promise since I never began a fight, our invalid [Madame C. had tuberculosis] said, "I'm real sorry girls that I'm not able to take a hand in that fight."

Then words, plenty of them, came to my assistance and said: "No, thank God! you are not able to take a hand; your hand has been lifted for the last time against poor insane women. The Lord has laid his hand upon you. You are going to die, do you know it? and that soon." And dying she was, the lingering death of the consumptive; yet with her gasping breath could express her regret at her inability to yet give me a blow!

After the fight was over, which was my last physical fight, I staggered back to my corner in such a wrathful, wicked state of mind as to be absolutely frightful even to recall. After a time two old ladies came and stood beside me and talked in a low voice of the outrage, and one of them said, "We two old women should tell Dr. Rogers [the superintendent] how this poor creature has been abused. She is dreadfully hurt for it is a dangerous thing to bruise a woman's breast." But they agreed that they didn't dare to report their attendants, and as a consequence no one outside was made acquainted with this ward secret.

Four years have passed, and I am yet at times a fearful sufferer from that painted, smiling fraud's brutality while she is still not without hope of again receiving employment at the Indiana State Hospital, and her companion in the outrage now occupies the position of attendant at an asylum in Kentucky and is as thoroughly an unfeeling and heartless girl as it has ever been my misfortune to meet. Yet it is more than probable her superintendent will read these disclosures doubtfully since no one knows any better than herself the art of deceiving those in authority.

On another occasion, when Anna Agnew was having severe loss of appetite and hallucinations about her food:

> . . . an attendant would hold my hands behind me, and another
> pour liquids down my throat, choking me so I must swallow or
> strangle. . . . Raw eggs, without a suspicion of salt, pepper or any-
> thing else to make them in the least palatable, were freely choked
> into my rebellious stomach. . . . I have seen those heartless girls fill
> a quart cup with a mixture of all the vegetables on the table, then
> salt and pepper and mustard by the spoonful, and after filling up the
> cup with vinegar, stir up the nasty mess and feed it by tablespoons-
> ful to some miserable wretch, crowding it down the unwilling
> throat⁻at the same time taunting and giggling over their misery.

Moral treatment included feeding patients who would not
eat. It did not, of course, include the abuses described. These abuses
occurred under the supervision of Madame C. and her supervisor, a
physician.

Villain

" 'I will break that woman's devilish will or I will break her damned
neck!' were the words spoken in my hearing by the physician in
charge of our ward." Anna Agnew did not mention the name of this
assistant physician, Dr. Walker, until near the end of the book. He
and Madame C. were described as working together and as being
like-minded about how patients should be treated: "Once she met
him as he was entering the door near me, and as he made this remark pointing to me with a backward turn of the thumb, 'There's a
fine subject for the dissecting table,' answered with a 'Ha! ha! she
is so!'"

Mrs. Agnew was referred to as "the devil" by the staff during a period of severe depression. Underlying her apparent hostility was delusional self-hatred which she described in painful detail but which many staff did not comprehend. Hostility, although not part of the definition of a major depressive episode, is not uncommon and usually represents a turning outward of ill feelings about oneself. Hell hath no fury like a woman depressed. Unfortunately, some staff responded in kind‑and much worse:

> I had gained the ill will of [Dr. Walker], and it was necessary for his reputation in that institution that I did not put into words my knowledge of his utter unworthiness of the position he occupied, and he ordered me transferred from the pleasant, cheerful ward upon which I had been . . . into a ward occupied exclusively by epileptics‑a class of patients of whom I stood in dreadful fear‑ hoping by such treatment that I would be so terrified as to become in reality the imbecile that he wrote to my sister he was pained to say I was fast becoming.

The fear of epileptics Anna Agnew expressed was not uncommon at the time or in prior ages. For example, epileptics in the Bible are described as being possessed by evil spirits. None of the anticonvulsants in use now was available. The epileptic patients committed to insane asylums had severe illness with frequent seizures and suffered other neurological problems, mental retardation, or psychiatric symptoms, all of which would appear frightening to a layperson. The fact that they were housed on a back ward reflects the hopelessness of their situation a century before antipsychotic medications became available to alleviate bizarre and destructive behavior. The sedatives and narcotic medications in use then would simply have made patients groggy.

Anna Agnew continued that she was on that ward for a year, beginning in May 1880. She returned to her former ward:

. . . with the same old calico dress hanging in tatters upon me, unchanged and unwashed, and with the same class of undergarments, changed each week for cleanliness but the quality or character not increased during the bitter cold winter of '80 and '81, and my greeting from the young lady (?) in charge of the ward (one of the *exclusives*) upon my return was: "Hello! Here comes the devil back!" My readers will please bear in mind that this treatment was in direct accordance with physician's orders concerning me. "Don't give that woman a change of dress until she asks for it," were his words, and I presume I would have worn that blessed calico frock until it dropped thread by thread off me since I came of stubborn old English stock on one side and Dutch on the other, only that I was weak enough in bodily strength one day to fall helpless in a congestive chill in which condition I was for an hour before I was allowed to be put to bed since, as the "young lady" said, when told by the doctor after he had examined me that I was a very sick woman and should have been in bed long before, "Well I couldn't tell whether she was really sick or just acting up!"

In consequence of this I was confined to my bed pretty sick, too, for several weeks and upon being taken up and ordered to dress myself in a complete new outfit consisting of comfortable clothing that all the preceding winter while I was shivering with cold had been stored away in the clothing room, my indignation got the better of my small stock of prudence, and I was suddenly possessed of a destructive spell, and tho' so weakened by sickness as not to be able scarcely to stand alone, I had sufficient strength to tear into bits four dresses as they were given me in succession for which I was punished by having my arms twisted by two strong attendants, discipline considered necessary to subdue an unruly patient. Before the fight was over the breakfast bell rang and I was driven into the dining-room clad in a single garment with the exception of my shoes and stockings and was seen in this condition by the engineer who came in before we were dismissed from the dining-room to attend to some necessary repairs.

The morning succeeding my transfer to the epileptic ward, the physician spoken of, in making his morning round, seated himself at a table just as I was in the act of placing a glass from which I had been drinking on the table and looking up at me said in a tantalizing tone of mock respect: "Good morning, Mrs. Agnew!" I took no notice of his salutation, but walked on toward my chair when he sprang to his feet with eyes flashing and face white with anger and said: "Don't you *dare* treat *me* with such contempt! Speak to me, madame!" and I, folding my arms, walked up to within striking distance and said: "You go to hell, sir!"

I hope he was satisfied with my speaking, and I trust my readers will consider that I was an insane woman at the time under his supposed protection and that the day previous he had grossly insulted me, the nature of which insult I will not soil this fair page in attempting to describe. . . . I am positive now that Dr. Rogers [the superintendent] was in entire ignorance of the shameful abuse to which I was subjected by that man who died trying to supercede him.

Anna Agnew was correct in her assessment of Dr. Joseph Rogers. He had written of moral treatment, "Pleasant social and material surroundings are necessary to general well being, and every effort is made to secure such as far as circumstances allow." With regard to seriously ill patients, he explained, "The system of restraint for the most violent patients is of the most humane and comfortable kind, is used as little as possible, never without the knowledge of the physician at the time, and only for a time. . . . Some form is indispensable, and these have proven themselves to be at the same time efficient and comfortable."

In a testimonial letter for Anna Agnew for her book in 1886, Rogers wrote, "I heartily wish your prospective literary venture may be a success. Let me say that among the many hundreds of my former patients I know of none so endowed by nature and culture with the ability to tell the story which your preface outlines. It will be a valuable contribution, not only to general literature, but to the library of the Alienist [psychiatrist]."

Anna Agnew described that her clothing was denied her. Annual reports of the hospital listed each patient's clothing by county of residence and who had paid for what. She had in storage at the hospital dresses, skirts, chemises, nightgowns, shawls, and underclothing brought with her on admission and had received from friends on July 23 and September 20, 1879, shoes, wrappers, sacques, yard goods, overshoes, and underclothing. The hospital billed the county for items provided to a patient and assumed the county would bill those responsible for the patient at home.

Much later Anna Agnew had opportunity to speak out to Madame C.:

> She had had her instructions, I presume, in regard to her treatment of me and proved herself fully competent to do any dirty bidding, and right well she followed her natural inclination until during this last administration she was delicately (?) hinted out of the institution. And as she was leaving [the hospital permanently] I staggered up of "my corner" and called after her: "Cleaning house on the fourth ward; good riddance of bad rubbish! There's more trash leaving this house this morning than ever left it at one time." She threw a startled, frightened glance over her shoulder as she sped down the hall, as much surprised, I imagine, as though a dead woman had sat up in her coffin and hurled those truths at her.

It was Anna Agnew's opinion that Dr. Walker was trying to become superintendent of the hospital. He died while working at the Indiana Hospital for the Insane as an assistant physician. Understandably, in view of her descriptions of his behavior, Anna Agnew reported his demise with less than sympathy:

And I hope most earnestly these two worthies [Madame C. and Dr. Walker] are not divided in death. Some enterprising disciple of Aesculapius should secure their anatomy, have them nicely articulated—dental arrangements—complete hers with gold fillings to similate [*sic*] nature. They should occupy the same office, grinning at each other through all eternity. "Male and female created he them." This letter was written during the first year of convalescence, and I offer no other apology for its bitterness.

John C. Walker had often been a center of controversy. His father had been a member of the state senate and was said to be the largest landowner in Indiana. Early in his career the younger Walker was successively editor of several newspapers around the state. Like his father he was interested in politics and was elected to the state legislature in 1853.

At this point his good fortune began to suffer reversal. Although he ran for lieutenant governor in 1855, he had to withdraw from that race because he was too young to hold the office. He ran unsuccessfully for Congress in 1858, and vigorously supported Democrat Stephen Douglas, the loser, in the presidential race against Republican Abraham Lincoln in 1860.

Walker was a "War Democrat" and joined the Union Army as an able drill officer and disciplinarian. As commander of the 35th Indiana Volunteers he served in campaigns in Tennessee and received a commendation from General Don Carlos Buell. He contracted typhoid fever and returned home to Indiana.

Governor Oliver P. Morton, a Lincoln Republican, dismissed him from military service. Walker fought his dismissal, finally moving to England where he lived until 1872. While there, by now in his early forties, he studied medicine at King's College, London, and married the daughter of a British naval officer. After returning to the United States, Dr. Walker studied at the Indiana Medical College and practiced in Shelbyville, Indiana, near Indianapolis. In 1879 he was appointed an assistant physician at the Indiana Hospital for the Insane, where he died from tuberculosis and diabetes in 1883.

The contemporary *History of Indianapolis and Marion County*, a publication of biographies supplied by the individuals discussed or by their friends, provided a laudatory appraisal of Dr. Walker's personality and activities. *Indiana in the Civil War Era* by Indiana historian Emma Lou Thornbrough presented a rather different assessment, one more in keeping with Anna Agnew's description of his behavior.

A vigorous campaign for the Indiana legislature occurred in 1862. Although Democrats vehemently criticized Republican Governor Morton, few of them actually favored the Confederacy. Many Democratic leaders actively worked against even the appearance of any such connection.

Both political parties had secret societies. One of these, composed of extremist Democrats, was the Sons of Liberty. Its principal tenet was devotion to states' rights, a major issue with the seceded Confederate states. Their leader was the infamous Clement Vallandigham, an Ohio Copperhead or Confederate sympathizer, who was banished behind Confederate lines and later escaped to Canada. He had proclaimed that the purpose of the Civil War was to free blacks and enslave whites.

John C. Walker was a member of the Sons of Liberty in Indiana, perhaps joining at the time of his conflict with Governor Morton. It was part of a bizarre plan that never came to fruition, and included obtaining arms from Confederate agents in Canada and formenting insurrection in Indiana and surrounding states. This association and the fact that many in the Sons of Liberty were arrested, tried, and jailed would explain Dr. Walker's move to England until well after the war.

When Anna Agnew encountered him, Walker's life had deteriorated from that of a promising young politician and military officer,
to that of a physician dying as he worked in a state mental hospital.
Temporarily redeemed by medical training and marriage in England,
he had reached the end of the line. It is not difficult to imagine that
he was embittered.

The able drill officer and disciplinarian, suffering illnesses that
would end his life, was now in charge of a ward of insane women.
He was even failing in an apparent attempt to be promoted to superintendent. His fight with Governor Morton presaged his rage at
a challenging female patient who did not know her place in his
scheme of things. Angry and embittered, the former drill officer
ignored her terrible melancholy. It was, however, part of his professional duty as a physician to try to understand patients and "to comfort always." He did neither.

Anna Agnew noted that the superintendent, Dr. Rogers, would
not have known of the behavior of Dr. Walker and Madame C. in
an institution housing hundreds of patients. Abusive staff found
adequate ways to avoid detection.

Rogers's life was much different than Walker's. Tuberculosis of
the spine had kept Joseph Goodwin Rogers bedfast from age twelve
to eighteen.In spite of his illness, he completed college studies during that time. After recovering, he read law for a year and then entered Bellevue Hospital Medical College in New York City, where
he was granted an M.D. degree in 1864.

As his father had done, he practiced in his hometown, Madison,
Indiana. Military service at the front lines was precluded by his
medical condition, but he became an acting assistant surgeon with
the army at the Madison General Hospital which served several
thousand wounded soldiers until the end of the Civil War.

He was superintendent of the Indiana Hospital for the Insane from
1879 to 1883, most of the years in which Anna was there. She noted
that during Rogers' four years as superintendent she had been too
depressed and miserable to respond to his repeated attempts at kind-

ness. She also mentioned his wife quite favorably. Hospital superintendents and their families were housed on the grounds of the
institutions they served. The wives served as "matrons" for the hospitals, performing small kindnesses for patients and generally acting rather like patient advocates. Their little sons playing on the
hospital grounds reminded her sadly of her own boys, whom she had
not seen since admission.

At the time of Anna Agnew's admission, the Indiana Hospital
for the Insane was the only such institution in the state. From 1883
to 1888 Dr. Rogers worked on a board of commissioners to develop
new hospitals and was superintendent of the first of these to open,
in Logansport. In 1898 he spoke at the state Conference of Charities and Corrections about the fact that the new hospitals, including two completed in 1890, were overflowing with patients and
asked for more facilities to be built. Rogers was honored nationally
as well as locally. In 1900 he was president of the American Medico-
Psychological Association, one of the forerunners of the American
Psychiatric Association.

Treatment, moral or immoral, in nineteenth century institutions
was conducted under public observation. Guests came to Seven
Steeples and other hospitals for the insane to "see the sights." The
custom of allowing anyone to visit institutions had begun as a
method of keeping conditions in hospitals under observation by the
general public. It had, however, deteriorated into entertainment.
Anna Agnew described with characteristic humor how patients
sometimes turned their own embarrassment back on the gaping
visitors:

> Could the general public the different classes of which visit such
> institutions with equally different motives, the professional sight
> seer, the philanthropist, the promiscuous excursion mob, or the
> select exclusive who occasionally honor the inmates with a super-
> cilious stare, know how frequently they are themselves outrageously
> duped by the poor crazy creature they have come to criticize, they

might not feel so comfortable. Scarcely a day passes without some such unpremeditated unadvertised exhibition being given. Particularly during the many state anniversaries, fairs, conventions, and many others of like character [in the state capital, Indianapolis] may such manifestations be expected and political campaigns furnish fun alive both to patients and visitors. And I can assure you that politics is not only a subject of conversation there [in the hospital] but is read of and understood, and party distinctions and lines are quite as closely drawn and pronounced as those [outside the hospital].

Our usher [for visitors] during the last campaign had as much as she could do to keep from betraying to visitors that they were the victims and that the patient quite as often understood themselves and the platform upon which they stood as did the smiling voter so very much amused [at patients' feigned confusion about politics]. Our attendants, too, all over the house frequently play patient, generally hanging lovingly on to some dudish sort of a chap whom they profess to recognize as some former lover, and several times quite touching scenes have been described by imaginative gushing reporters from some of our most reputable papers. . . .

During the last presidential campaign I had a large picture of our president hanging in my room plainly visible to visitors passing through the ward. I was entirely well then but still retained my room on the ward and sat there the greater part of the time sewing. My attendants and the usher told me they would hold themselves in readiness to at any time fall in with any joke I wished to play, and often visitors would stop at my door attracted by my candidate's picture and would talk in subdued voices of the "quiet looking patient sitting there sewing so intently" and Alice—our usher—would say with a sly mischievous look at me, "Yes, poor woman, she sits there most of her time generally quiet, but this fall she is greatly excited at times over politics, and is as you see a democrat, but she don't like folks to stare at her so we had better move on." One day during September of '84 a gentleman came in alone with Alice, and just before reaching my room she gave a peculiar significant little ahem! And I heard her say, "oh, Cleveland, of course! She has his picture. Just glance in as we pass as she is excited today and at such times is considered dangerous." I sprang up, ran my hands through my short hair which was just sufficiently curly at that sort of treatment to stand "looking seven ways for Sunday" and was ready for inspection. He glanced in with a short merry "ha! ha! So she is still a democrat? That speaks well for the democracy!" and I recognized even by that slight glimpse a resemblance to Cleveland and started on the jump after him! If you could have witnessed that race down the short hall to the turn which he rounded like a locomotive, then down the long hall to the door out of which he sprang as the attendant, who ran ahead pretending to be terribly frightened for the man's safety, opened it. Just as he reached the door I struggled away from the usher who was pretending with the greatest difficulty to hold me while she screamed to the brave fellow, "run, run! My goodness, man don't let her catch you," and [I] grabbed him by the coat collar crying, "no, sir! Grover you don't escape me this time! I've got you!" The horrified expression in that man's eyes will never leave me as he looked back over his shoulders and sprang out into the hall banging the door after him! Cleveland made a pretty good presidential race but not to compare with his prototype trying to escape from a crazy admirer

In reality, public visitors were no laughing matter. When she recovered, Anna Agnew became a strong advocate for patient privacy. The following appeared as the next to last chapter of the book and in the *Indianapolis Herald,* February 20, 1886, almost a year after Anna Agnew had left Indiana Hospital for the Insane. In the newspaper, her reference to herself in the letter is printed as "Mrs. ———."

A TOUCHING APPEAL

We hope every member of the Indiana Legislature will read the article in today's Herald entitled, "A Touching Appeal." The writer is a lady of unusual intelligence, who passed several years in the Indianapolis Asylum for the Insane, and was at last completely restored, as her strongly written appeal abundantly proves. The custom of admitting curiosity seekers into the institution had its origin in the suspicion of maltreatment, and is at last reflection on the efficacy and probity of the asylum officials. It is as much as to say, if the people don't believe we are attending to our duties, let them come and see for themselves, and nine-tenths of the opened-mouthed starers who visit the institution have no interest beyond mere idle curiosity; a common phase of the milder forms of insanity is morbid sensitiveness, and the effect of being glowered at by strangers can not be better described than it is in the article of "Non Compos Mentis," who has felt it in all its accumulated terrors.

EDITOR.

To the Honorable Gentlemen of the Indiana Legislature:

It has been impressed upon my mind, since my discharge from the hospital for the insane—as a patient—that it is a duty I owe to humanity to make an appeal to the legislature for a law prohibiting the promiscuous visiting at that institution, and were it in my power to make you understand the positive torture many of those peculiarly unfortunate people suffer from the mere presence of the throngs of impertinent morbid curiosity seekers from whom there is no escape in the wards of their prison I am sure my attempt in their behalf will not be in vain. I use the word prison advisedly, and without intending the slightest reflections upon the management. "Bolts and bars" are but trifles compared with the mental torture endured by many of those miserable, self-convicted criminals, and suggest only the hope of rest and security from fancied persecution. Poor afflicted victims! gathering a fearful harvest, not alone of their own sowing, tossed and tortured, and driven by a fate worse than death! Such, indeed, need an asylum, and such all institutions for the insane should be, and the "bolts and bars" that lock them and their terrible burden of misery within should assuredly lock without those who would curiously gaze upon without the slightest appreciation of their suffering the unhappy inmates. People are not insensible when insane, either to praise, censure or ridicule, and though I am far from charging all who visit the wards of the insane as being actuated by morbid curiosity, I do claim that there are but few exceptions among the inmates who do not resent such as intrusions; even the visits of relatives are not always a kindness. I know this in all its horrors; for three years almost I sat in one spot in the same old rocking chair, on the fourth ward of the hospital for the insane, fighting a battle with the Almighty, feeling I had no right to live, but not allowed to die, hoping and praying to choke to death at every bite I ate, yet forced to swallow food. Hating and cursing the sun that it shone and the flowers that they would bloom. A self-convicted criminal, answering at the judgment seat, my conscience, for every idle word or wicked thought, and yet as though my cup was not already full, I was outraged and tortured by the idle, unfeeling comments of careless people, sometimes strangers, often former friends, who I am sure, now, could not realize how they hurt me, but most frequently of persons whom I had formerly only known the existence of, who would not have dared presume to speak to, or of me before I "went crazy." Even now, in every nerve of my body, I realize the horror that seemed to take possession of my very soul as I would hear some one asking to see me, as a noisy crowd on "an excursion to Indianapolis," and bound to see the sights, was passing through the wards, and the answer of my attendant, "that's her settin' down there in the corner, but she's too mean to speak to anyone, but go try her if you want to." At such times I have held up my poor helpless hands, and watched the goose flesh gather and stand upon my arms, and felt the cold chills creep over me as I waited and shivered in anticipation of the remarks sure to follow. "Can that be Mrs. Agnew?" "Don't she ever speak?" "Does she always sit there?"

"Why, dear me, isn't it queer? she used to do so-and-so, and she used to be such-and-such" and all I, poor miserable wretch, could do, was to wish the whole world,—particularly the female world—had one neck and I had the power to strangle the life out of it. Oh, how bitterly I resented such cruelty, and I am sure mine is not an exceptional case in this respect, though certainly my complete recovery is an exceptional one, and I am happy in being able to assure those so unfortunate as to have dear ones needing the protection of such place, that they need feel no uncertainty of such receiving the kindest attention from the officers in your hospital for insane, and when leaving there myself after seven years, I felt indeed that I was leaving my home. With this exception, which lies within your power, gentlemen of the legislature, to remedy, the Hospital for the Insane of Indiana, embodies humanity in its truest sense.

Very sincerely,
"NON COMPOS MENTIS"

This favorable view of hospital staff was written after Dr. Walker had died and Madame C. had left the institution. Mrs. Agnew had come under the care of much different physicians and staff. She did not criticize the superintendents and lamented that "politics is permitted to lay its blighting hand upon this the noblest of state charities." The hospital, located in the capital city of Indianapolis, became a battleground for politics in the 1880s. Staff positions were often awarded on the basis of political loyalty. Superintendents changed with each new governor. Finally, in 1889 a bipartisan Board of State Charities was established by the legislature to oversee state institutions.

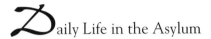aily Life in the Asylum

Anna Agnew gave an excellent, detailed account of daily life at the Indiana Hospital for the Insane. This is rather unusual in nineteenth-century memoirs of patients pleading for asylum reform in that her account is not primarily polemical and provides details about mundane occurrences in the lives of patients. This account, like many in the book, was from a letter she wrote during hospitalization that was saved for her by the recipient:

> This place reminds me of a great clock, so perfectly regular and smooth are its workings, and certainly any latent [tendency of a patient for] order stands a good chance of development here. The system is perfect; our bill of fare is excellent, and varied, as in any well regulated family and especially, we have good bread. We retire at the ringing of the telephone at eight o'clock, and an hour later, there's darkness and silence that can almost be felt all over this vast building, excepting an occasional piercing cry from some restless soul not yet under the kindly influence of night medicine. And the silence is scarcely disturbed by the light, careful step of the night watch, as she makes her half hour rounds. Flitting quickly along, she throws the penetrating light of her tiny lantern into each room through the elliptical openings in the panels, ready at the slightest sound from the inmates to respond with kindly inquiry of "What's wanting there?" And as I lay there, hour after hour, thinking—for I

am yet a poor sleeper—my mind goes longingly back to the past; way back to my childhood, stopping here and there to cull a flower from some sweet memory. . . .

After a while though, the ting-a-ling-ling of the ward telephone says, "Get up, it is five o'clock in the morning," and the same old routine begins again; and I'd like you to find a busier or as funny a scene, as an early morning on an insane ward—women in all stages of deshabille—are running here and there, fussing and spatting over disputed articles of wearing apparel, in some cases monopolizing their own and their neighbors' outfit. Plenty of time is given us to make our not elaborate toilet. Plenty of soap and water, hot and cold. An abundance of clean towels, combs and brushes; and when the breakfast bell summons us to the dining-room, no one need complain of the breakfast that greets us—though in the winter sometimes we do get fearfully tired of the perfect regularity with which a certain meat stew makes its appearance. Almost any luxury (?) becomes sort of monotonous after six or seven years' indulgence, and we earnestly hoped last winter when the kitchen burned, that its valuable recipe was consumed, but was informed by our careful druggist that he could furnish a duplicate, since all valuable concoctions, such as that stew, are religiously preserved. This last paragraph was an after-thought, not included in my letter to my sister.

After breakfast every "lady" who is able and willing for duty goes to work, every body knowing exactly what to do, and none daring to infringe upon her neighbors' territory, or fancied right, for I assure you they are quite as tenacious of their rights, and far more so of their dignity than many of their sane sisters outside the bars— after a while the ward is completely put to rights, and in splendid order, too, without the slightest disagreement or disorder, with only an occasional "come, come, 'ladies,' not quite so noisy!" from the attendant. But quite frequently some "servant" will give an impertinent reply to some important "mistress of this house, I'll have you understand!"—said mistress, as is frequently the case in the best regulated families, having gotten up out of sorts, or as we in asylum par-

lance say, "a little off,"—when presto, change! And scrubbing buck-
ets, mops, broom-sticks and what not! Any thing that serves for a
weapon, comes into active use, to say nothing of tongues! But unlike our sane sisters outside, we can't order our sassy servants to "pack
up their traps and leave, and we will do our work ourselves." No,
indeed! "servants" and "mistresses" are on a complete level here,
but generally, on our ward we are a quite orderly crowd.

Women in the nineteenth century were adept at needlework, as
was Anna Agnew, and the hospital used their skills to produce ser-
viceable garments and linens for inmates and to keep the hands of
patients busy. Indeed, it was an early version of occupational therapy.
Keeping patients productively employed dates back at least to the
beginning of the asylum movement in eighteenth-century Europe,
if not to antiquity. Then, as now, such useful occupations as sewing
and gardening were seen as therapeutic, and at one time there was
a farm associated with the Indiana Hospital for the Insane, a common feature of asylums. In the twentieth century occupational
therapy became a profession requiring two years of postgraduate
training covering much broader areas of therapy and theory than
the simple activities of nineteenth-century asylums.

In nineteenth-century America such activities of patients saved
money for the hospital as was duly noted in the annual reports to
the state legislature. Employment of patients by the hospital was
made illegal nationally in the late twentieth century in order to
avoid exploitation of patients' labor.

Anna Agnew described the sewing-room that she attended as her
condition improved as follows:

> The sewing-room of the institution is esteemed an oasis in their
> otherwise monotonous life. It is a large room on the fourth floor,

extending over the entire center building, and its high ceiling and immense windows make it a splendid and cheerful looking room. There are a number of regularly employed sewing girls under the supervision of a forewoman, and it is wonderful the amount of sewing that is done there monthly. Dresses, as one item, running up well into the hundreds, and all other garments worn by women in the same proportion, besides the regular weekly or monthly requisitions of the ward and official departments of bedding, towels, napkins and table-cloths, including also curtains necessary, all through this large building.

The patients are divided into two classes—home supplied and state or county patients—and many of the friends of those supplied at home prefer to furnish the material and have themselves charged with the making by the state. So one may imagine the hundreds of yards of material used there monthly.

Going to the sewing-room to assist is not obligatory upon any patient. But the messenger from there at 9 a.m. very rarely opens the door of any ward, and calls "ladies for the sewing-room" without a ready response from some half a dozen or more anxious to get to work. And soon after nine a wonderful big sewing bee is in full swing.

Imagine, if you can, such a clatter of tongues! For woman will talk, sane or insane, and busy fingers as well as tongues fly, and occasionally some singer (?) will tune up and numerous others will join in, each singing her own particular tune, or no tune at all, and some body else will for variety swear until the atmosphere is blue, while over there in the patching corner several old cronies are enjoying a choice dish of gossip, discussing their ward secrets that they have been cautioned strictly by their attendants not to tell at the sewing-room, but which they invariably do tell, very much after the manner of their sane sisters.

And so the wonderful machine moves on day after day smoothly as well regulated works always do when the "master mechanic" is at the same time kind hearted as well as level-headed. The sewing-room, from its importance to the institution on account of its work, also being an important curative factor in the treatment of the insane since by this means their thoughts are directed from themselves thus inducing forgetfulness of personal sorrow by giving employment to their hands.

Anna Agnew had a penetrating eye for the individual idiosyncrasies of those around her; her observations of the human aspects of both patients and staff are the real substance of her book and provide the most interesting reading for us today. When she entered the Indiana Hospital for the Insane the population of patients there was about equally divided between men and women. They were housed in separate wards and, ultimately, in separate buildings after the Women's Building was constructed. Ages ranged from under ten to over eighty, with most patients in their twenties, thirties, or forties. About 12 percent of women were married women aged forty to fifty, as was Anna Agnew. Eighty percent of patients were American born, as was she, 10 percent German born, and 5 percent born in Ireland. No mention is made in hospital statistics of African Americans although the list of religious affiliations indicates a few African Methodists. One-fourth of the patients had a "good common school" education like Anna Agnew, but half could "read and write only." At the extremes were some who were illiterate and others who were college educated or professionals.

She had been diagnosed with "acute mania." That this represented many diagnostic categories now used is indicated by the fact that 41 percent of patients were given this diagnosis. Two-thirds of patients had been ill less than one year, one-fifth less than one month. There were just over 50,000 psychiatric patients in 150 institutions, most of them public, in the United States and its territories. This was the only insane asylum in Indiana, a state that at the time had a population of two million.

The institution was a village in itself. The villagers had to get acquainted, get along, and find friends as well as enemies. Anna Agnew wrote:

> I believed the patients generally liked me, at any rate I was made the recipient of a many a tale of woe and petitioned for sympathy . . .
>
> I still continued the confidential friend of the majority of the patients, and I allowed them free access to my room [after her recovery] when there myself, making but one single proviso, they were *not to cry*, I had enough of that sort of thing to do myself. One poor little woman, who did nothing else for about three months after she came, told me after her recovery, what a temptation my room used to be to her at times; that often she could scarcely restrain her impulse to rush in there and demolish every thing there, myself included, because I would not allow her to come to me with her everlasting "I want to go home!" I, too, wanted with all my heart to go home and was in a condition to go but my misery in this regard was not of a sort that loved company; we were good friends though through it all, and I helped her get ready to go home when after only a few months stay, her husband gladly came for her.

Anna Agnew discussed altercations among hostile patients including some threats of attack on herself. Although she could be quite assertive at such times, she did not express anger at the patients, themselves, for behavior that was the product of illness:

> Insane persons seem naturally suspicious and generally are jealous, and the fact of me being presented at the time I began at the sewing-room with a key to use at my discretion was the means of my receiving one morning, when assisting my attendant with the

morning work, a blow upon my head by an iron mop stick in the hands of an infuriated "mistress of this house, I'll have you understand," that made the blood fly and laid me senseless for a few moments. I had just fitted my key in the lock of the clothing-room, when I heard, rather than felt the blow. Such things *will* sometimes occur and often give rise to sensational newspaper articles of "patients in our insane asylum being allowed to batter the life out of each other, a state of affairs needing investigation," etc. etc. Patients do sometimes kill each other, and the attendants are not to blame, are at times powerless to prevent it, since it comes so suddenly; and it were well for the public to charitably reflect before deciding against the management of any such institution since a very slight fire will, under encouraging circumstances, sometimes smoke considerably. It is the "ward secrets" hidden, particularly, and especially from the superintendent and physicians, that I am contending against.

Anna Agnew sometimes described other patients' bizarre behavior with gentle amusement but without condescension:

As the officers of the new administration made their first appearance in the wards one old lady, who had been a patient for twenty years, therefore witnessing several such changes and by virtue of staying considered herself "one of the family," said with a contemptuous look as one of the new comers was making his first official round, "Damned upstart, he had better get one of us to show him how to run this she-bang!" Everybody in the asylum knew "Aunt Betty" and her tongue, and it was considered the part of wisdom not to question her right to remarks, neither was it always safe to reply to them. But she was a reasonable old lady and like many of her sane sisters a little politic, too. So she was not long in recognizing the worthiness of the new administration.

In another letter of later date I wrote:

You have no idea of the celebrities we have here in our board-ing-house. First and eldest is "Aunt Betty" B, who is everybody's "Aunt Betty" when at her normally insane self but at her times of excitement—which are quite frequent is "Mrs. Elizabeth B.! I thank you! Don't you dare Aunt Betty me! And I'm no pauper I'll have you to understand! I could buy you and all your kit if you were black! And it's none of your infernal business if I have been here twenty years! You don't pay my bills!" On her annual or semi-annual "tears," in hospital slang, she demolishes every thing perishable in her "old curiosity shop," as her room with its miscellaneous collection of odds and ends may well be called, and as she goes tearing up and down the hall with her thin, straggling gray hair, which she is everlast-ingly trying to comb, flying in all directions, her clothing hanging in tatters upon her, and her feet thrust into the doctor's old slip-pers. Often she looks but little like the tidy, ruffled-aproned, good tempered "Aunt Betty" that everybody knows and is kind to. . . .

. . . and "Mrs. President Hays" has boarded here for ten years, and all this time her husband reigns at Washington, and she can't imag-ine why he does not allow her to go there too and take her rightful position as first lady of the land. Of course she can't see why, poor woman! And I am afraid she never will understand why this is thus, tho' by birth and education she is not unfitted to such a position.

About the handsomest old lady and important . . . I ever saw is the "Autocrat" of our dining-room, Auntie H. She is employed at an annual salary of eighty millions to superintend the workings of the universe, as pertains to earthly affairs, but does not aspire to heavenly matters. Her headquarters are here and her agents, tried and true, are scattered through the "uttermost parts of the earth," and she receives and responds to their constant reports by telephone. As a consequence of such extended territory and the importance of the communications, her telephone, otherwise mouth, is never shut. She talks from morning til night and all night and the next day!

And she is quite as extensively married as she is otherwise burdened with care. To her certain knowledge she has been married seventeen times, and is the anxious mother of two hundred and fifty children of her own besides a whole lot of step-children and grand-children.

These patients obviously had grandiose delusions. One likely diagnosis is mania. Another possibility in the late nineteenth century was paresis, the late stage of syphilis, for which there was no cure seventy years before antibiotics. Because of the years that elapsed between infection and the onset of psychiatric symptoms, it was not even recognized as a stage of syphilis until about 1900. Patients with paresis were a significant portion of patients in asylums at the time. They often appeared manic before the gradual mental and physical deterioration of their illness set in. That Aunt Betty had been there twenty years makes paresis a less likely diagnosis for her. A patient with paresis would have died within a few years.

In other letters Anna Agnew had written while in the hospital, saved by family and friends and given to her after she left the asylum, she had written:

Persons in general can have no idea of the warm personal attachments formed among this unfortunate class. Once during my second year in the asylum an old German woman on our ward was reported at the point of death and upon no account was she to be given water to drink. She had been one of the silent sort, too, scarcely ever speaking to any one, but as I went into her room just at twilight, she said, "Oh good lady, shust one drink for God's sake!" I said, "Mrs. C. they say water will kill you!" "No, no," she cried, "I will die without." And so I made her promise not to tell and gave her a tin cupful. She drank as tho' famished and sank back on her pillow gasping, "so goot, so goot, so goot!" The next morning her bed was vacant. And I did not know until four years after but that my cup of water killed her.

One day after having attained to the dignity of a "trusty," having keys of my own, I thank you, I was going through the other division from ours when some one caught me around the neck crying, "The good laty, I not forget, I not forget, I never vill!" and there was my dead old friend, bright as a lark! The happiest old lady in the ward! But alas! Never to come from under her cloud. Yet she did not forget the cup of cold water given in violation of the rules!

Associations could be strong among patients. Another friendship with a less happy outcome was described elsewhere in the book:

Soon after my admission I formed the acquaintance of a woman of unusual intelligence, an inmate of an adjoining ward, who I frequently met when out walking for exercise. We had many thoughts in common and congenial literary taste, but directly opposite in our ideas regarding the sinfulness of suicide. I openly expressed my sincere belief that since we were brought into the world independent of our wish or will, we had a perfect right to chose whether or no we stay here, after life hath lost its charms and was to us simply an impatiently borne burden!

We had one last talk together the day upon which the new building [the Women's Building] was given over into the hands of the state trustees, and the crowds of people and band music attendant upon the occasion seemed to worry her dreadfully. As usual in our conversations, we talked of suicide together with the question of the possible return of departed spirits and their communication with their friends.

During our conversation she said: "Well, my friend, you and I have had pleasant, enjoyable times together here, but I must believe that suicide is the unpardonable sin! Since for this there is no repentance.

So, if I should kill myself tonight, I believe I should go right straight to hell! I don't presume in that case I would be permitted to return, neither do I suppose you would care to receive a visit from a lost soul! And should I be so unspeakably happy as to find myself in heaven I might not be inclined to leave there even for a short time. But just as surely as spirits are permitted to return, when I go away, I will return to you!"

As we parted in the hall separating our wards, she said good-by! She was not a patient requiring close attention during the night, and in the morning her dead body was found suspended stiff and stark in her lonely little room! And her soul, pure and white, I am certain, had found the mystery of all its sad questionings.

Did she return to me? Time and again! Not with the stooping, fragile body and care-stamped face of my departed friend! But with the springing, buoyant step and bright laughing face of her early married life so often talked of when she counted not past years by their tears and dreamed of no hereafter without its joyous hopes.

A genuine belief that suicide is a sin does not prevent severely depressed patients from committing suicide. They already believe themselves to be so evil as to be beyond any salvation. Suicide in an episode of major depressive disorder is especially tragic because recovery is likely. When their illness is in remission, patients who have been depressed do not commit suicide.

Anna Agnew's independence of mind about religious as well as other matters expressed itself elsewhere in the book. Not only did she come to disdain her husband's "unspotted old Irish Presbyterian family," but she also lost her faith in her own apparently traditional upbringing. She mentioned in a letter that there was one church in Moscow, Ohio, when she was growing up. It was Methodist. This denomination was prominent in that area in the early nineteenth century. A Methodist pastor in Moscow married her and her husband.

In discussing the fact that she had no intention of blaming any person for being a *cause* of her insanity, she wrote:

> I place the responsibility exactly where it belongs. The Almighty controls such matters. We are his creatures, utterly helpless in his hands. And, however we may struggle and grow desperate in our efforts to reconcile the directly opposite attributes, those of a kind and merciful Father, who pities our infirmities, who never willingly afflicts his children, whose cross is not too heavy to be borne, with the same Father who speaks us into existence, bearing within us traits that must ripen into a harvest fearful beyond words to express. And, though his promises are that we shall not be tried beyond our strength, that the back shall be fitter for the burden, *does* desert us in our extremity.
>
> Let those who have never thus been so fearfully tried reconcile these inconsistencies if they can; and love the One who embodies them if they choose. I do not care to enter into a controversy of the matter; but at the same time do claim the right to question his methods and the instruments used.
>
> My stock originally of the commodity, unquestioning faith, was limited to a small amount; and years and experience have not increased it. I have learned by bitter sorrow the fallacy of trusting even the promises of God. Implicit faith in anybody or any thing is a thing of the past; and its absence is not greatly regretted. I believe I am happier since; certainly I am more content.
>
> I remember that I used to dwell with horror upon the bible-inspired thought of being left to myself! Given up! And numerous other terrible threatenings. And no thought gave me such horror as the possibility of endless torment after death in spite of earnest effort to live correctly. Such doubts and fears trouble me no longer; for of this I am certain, this life nor the hereafter holds nothing for me worse than the past! The very bitterest cup that malignant fate

holds for mortals, I have drank to the last drop! Friendless and alone, I have fought this demon, insanity! and have come out strengthened for whatever the future holds for me.

I have passed through a furnace of affliction such as few are called upon to endure; and whether the dross in my nature be purified or not there's no depth of misery I have not sounded. And where is the theologian who can successfully refute my sincere belief that insanity is the *real hell* spoken of in the Bible?

This was written after all that had happened to her before and during hospitalization, including her experience of the depressive symptoms of delusional guilt and hopelessness. Severely depressed individuals not infrequently lose their faith, at least as long as they are depressed. Conversely, to some a depression, or more especially recovery, might strengthen belief and be perceived as a religious experience. Anna Agnew, while eschewing traditional religion, saw her experience as strengthening.

She was preparing at the time of the writings just quoted to engage in what would be extremely unpleasant divorce proceedings. The interaction with her husband in his few visits to the hospital had been increasingly hostile. For many in the nineteenth century Presbyterian belief was often popularly interpreted to mean that God predetermines everything that happens, and we should accept both good and bad as God's will. Subscribing to older doctrines about predestination, some thought that God chose in the beginning who would be saved and who would be damned. Anna Agnew seemed to refer to this when she wrote of "endless torment after death in spite of earnest effort to live correctly."

In another part of the book, angry that a physician in Vincennes involved in her commitment to the hospital had advised that she be sent to the penitentiary, she wrote: "If the Christian standard of the Presbyterian Church be maintained, of which at that time this man was an elder, he is a subject for Presbyter investigation. And is not *perjury* punishable in the civil courts?"

She was likely referring also to a hellfire-and-damnation nineteenth-century religious perspective. Her Methodist upbringing would have involved religious "revival" meetings, many of which took place in Moscow, Ohio, when she was young. That she was familiar with revival meetings is indicated elsewhere in the book such as in her discussion of playing the piano for other patients in the hospital to sing the old hymns that many loved. This resulted in several patients mimicking half-seriously the rousing style of the revival preaching that resulted in requests, the "altar call," for people to come to the altar to confess their sins and their desire to change their lives.

Religion was a serious matter in nineteenth-century America. Historians Roger Finke and Rodney Stark have described some of the denominational differences: Methodists and Presbyterians in the Midwest had many an argument about "predestination" (Presbyterian) versus "free will" (Methodist), the belief that one's fate is not predetermined; Presbyterians belonged to a more established, sedate church and Methodists to a church likely to emphasize emotional outdoor "camp meetings." Such religious differences might well have been a source of conflict between Anna Agnew and her husband, although she was able to convince him to have their marriage performed by a Methodist minister in her hometown.

More in line with what would be expected of Methodist preaching of the time would be references to frightened sinners screaming as the devil carried them off. To Anna Agnew that included the "horror" of a "bible-inspired thought of being left to myself! Given up! And numerous other terrible threatenings." Similar views in some of those around her during her illness would hardly have been comforting especially if her illness itself were seen as sin worthy of the devil's attentions.

It is much easier to see suffering as God's will if it is happening to someone else. Perhaps some well-meaning family or friends had expressed such views, tragically not uncommon in somewhat modified form in those comforting the sick even today. Anna Agnew's picture of herself is reminiscent of the situation of Job and his less than helpful friends. Unlike Job, however, she was unable to "reconcile the inconsistencies" between a kind and loving God and her own experiences of suffering.

Religious services were often a part of moral therapy. Early in her hospitalization, after the altercations with her Presbyterian relatives and physician about her admission and while still quite depressed, Anna Agnew noted:

> I had not been there long until I noticed that certain patients in each ward were requested, or rather expected, to go to religious services held in the chapel, and it caused very anxious thoughts on my part. I was not inclined then to disobey any of the rules but most certainly did not intend to go to church. So, I asked Dr. Hester if I would ever be compelled to go? "No," he said, "certainly not; you are unsettled enough now on points of theology. I will never force your inclination in that direction; neither do I think any party succeeding us will do so. But I certainly hope some time the Lord may so incline your heart that you will go willing.
>
> I don't know at all if the doctor is himself piously inclined or not but as I answered, "Oh, the Lord has nothing at all to do with me! We have parted company long since!" he said, "So you are able to live independently of the Lord, are you? Well, that's something I don't care to try."

Religious historian Ann Taves observed that theologians of various perspectives and researchers in the newly developing field of psychology engaged in numerous discussions in the late nineteenth century. Popular views of religion and psychology included speculations about human behavior that took different paths from traditional religion. One of these, spiritualism, was mentioned by Anna Agnew in her discussion of the suicide of her friend in the hospital:

> I am not a believer in any form of spiritualism that I have ever read of or heard spoken of, but I have a theory that insane persons are brought directly under spiritual influence not to be explained. My father [who had been dead several years] was with me constantly for months! So sensible was I of his presence that I often put out my hand, thinking surely I would touch him. But the time came when he said, " I am going to leave you now, my daughter, and I am not coming back again!" And from that time I was indeed alone!

As Taves noted, spiritualists blurred the boundary between popular psychological theory and the various spiritual "awakenings" that characterized religious life in America at the time. Anna Agnew's contemporaries often consulted psychics or mediums to put them in touch with departed loved ones. Mary Todd Lincoln was among those who did so. The ghost of Abraham Lincoln hovers over her in a tintype taken by a spiritualist photographer.

Anna Agnew experienced her father's spirit as her protector. However, with spiritualism, as with nineteenth-century Protestant views, she remained a skeptic.

CHAPTER SIX

$\mathcal{L}$ooking Back, Looking Forward

Like American society in the late nineteenth century, the practice of psychiatry was changing. No one quite knew where either was going. Later in her hospitalization Anna Agnew was fortunate to have some physicians who returned to some of the better principles of eighteenth-century moral treatment while beginning to see treatment in a perspective more like that of the twentieth century.

Dr. Walker was replaced by Dr. Andrew J. Thomas. Of the change, Anna said:

> Death had removed my enemy, and he was succeeded by Dr. Thomas, a gentleman who soon made his presence and influence felt. . . .Through his kindness my surroundings had already been made more comfortable, and though keenly appreciating his attentions, I had not yet been able in the slightest to respond to them.

Dr. Thomas was an assistant physician at the Indiana Hospital for the Insane from 1879 to 1890. Born in Mississippi in 1840, he graduated from the University of Missouri. After what he would have called the War between the States, he traveled north because of financial reverses caused by the war. He graduated from Jefferson Medical College, Philadelphia, in 1867 and began his practice of medicine in Oaktown, Indiana. Later he moved to nearby Vincennes where he was elected auditor of Knox County and was editor of the

Vincennes Sun. The newspaper failed financially, and he moved to Indianapolis to work at the hospital. He was later superintendent of the Southern Indiana Hospital for the Insane at Evansville. Anna Agnew did not mention specifically whether she had known him in Vincennes but described him favorably in the book:

One morning as he was making his usual morning rounds, he asked my attendant to bring him a chair, saying as he seated himself by my rocking-chair, "You need not wait here, I want to have a talk with Mrs. Agnew." Good heavens, a talk with me! I was terribly frightened. No one ever talked with me; they only talked at and about me, and I knew not what to expect, but his manner was kind and he began, "I want to talk to you this morning about that terrible night medicine to which you have become such a slave (a preparation of chloral given to produce sleep).

"Why," he said. "when I examined the report of the night watch this morning, I was absolutely shocked at the amount of that miserable stuff given you last night. Do you know that the last dose given you would have killed me, strong man as I am; and I presume it had only the effect of confusing you, making you drunk. Now then, listen to me. That medicine won't kill you, but its continued use will make you a miserable imbecile, and you don't want to become that; you want to get well and go home to your family. Now there's no doubt about your will power to stop this right straight off, and I want your promise this morning that you will never again ask the night watch for another single drop. Once you make this promise, and I believe you are just the woman to keep your word, and in return I pledge you my word that I will instruct the night watch to give you all you wish if you do ask for it."

And he said farther, " I must tell you that you are undertaking a great struggle. It will be far worse than the drunkard stopping drink. You may be reduced to the weakness of an infant, but we will all help you, give you our sympathy, and sometime you will thank me for my effort to save you."

I promised him I would try, and I succeeded. I doubt that prayers of mine would avail to shower down blessings upon his head, but certainly if in the present or future my restored intellect and sound body adds happiness to any friend of mine, they will join me in my sincere affection and gratitude to him. In my extremity I had a friend. I will not attempt a description of my agony of mind and body before the victory was complete; the recollections are too painful.

Those who have fought and conquered the opium habit may have some conception of the state of complete prostration to which I was reduced. And my sufferings have made me more tolerant in my condemnation of any weakness of poor humanity. Afterward I asked permission of the doctor to read Luther Benson's *Fifteen Years in Hell* feeling that I could fully sympathize with the author in his attempt at describing his feelings when fighting the demons of delirium tremens.

At another point Anna Agnew explained:

Night medicine is a preparation of chloral, and it was given me the first night I spent in this place, and has been continued every night since, excepting as occasionally it would occur to Dr. Walker that probably I might be deriving some comfort from its use, and he would discontinue its use for a time.

At such periods I was wild and wretched in the extreme! Not that it served its purpose with me—that of producing sleep! It simply kept me from continuous thought, and kept me in bed too, since its effect upon me was to make me drunk—so that I would fall helpless upon the floor, unable, without the assistance of the night watch, to get up again. But deprived of it, all night long I would walk the floor wringing my hands, with my familiar spirit ever by my side, with its horrible accusations repeated, and met by denial on my part until worn out, and desperate, I would make confession of sins, only slightly conceived of in my real mind. Then would follow the taunt-ing voice: "Why don't you kill your worthless self, then? Why don't you? Others have done this, why not you? You don't dare to! You shall not! You shall live, and live! You shall never die!"

And all this time just outside my door, where on moonlight nights I could plainly see it, standing upon the table was the night medi-cine, which if I could only, Oh God! If I only could get it once, alone! I could drink myself to death and forgetfulness of all this misery. But at such times not one drop could I beg, even to scatter these desper-ate thoughts. All I could do was to stand at the door, with my face pressed through the openings, gazing at my hope of nepenthe and cursing that villainous doctor!

By the time of Anna Agnew's hospitalization, a few of the medi-cations that would be used in the twentieth century were available: salicylates (compounds similar to aspirin), morphine injections for pain, and bromide salts and chloral hydrate for sedation. Warner has described the development of chloral hydrate through labora-tory research in Germany. In what would become standard practice in pharmacology, it was tried in laboratory animals and then in clini-cal trials in patients. Its action, sedation, was predicted on the basis of the scientific knowledge of the time. The predicted action, but not the hypothetical basis for that action, proved correct. Its pro-posed metabolism in the body, predicted in 1869, turned out to be erroneous, but it did help patients to sleep. These fortuitous guesses would often determine what new medications would be tried until the more accurate predictions of molecular biology in the late twen-tieth century.

Chloral hydrate, like most other sedatives and alcohol, has the potential for producing tolerance (larger and larger doses are needed to achieve the same effect) and physical dependence (when suddenly stopped a characteristic withdrawal syndrome occurs). Tolerance and physical dependence, alone, in the absence of the other symptoms of addiction, are simply related to the pharmacological properties of the medication.

Anna Agnew experienced the equivalent of delirium tremens seen in alcohol withdrawal. Her physicians apparently understood the potential for symptoms of withdrawal. As she described it, Dr. Walker used them in a callous, punitive manner while Dr. Thomas showed professional and compassionate regard for his patient.

What was not realized at the time was the importance of detoxification, the gradual tapering of doses to prevent most of the withdrawal symptoms. The danger of not tapering sedative medication gradually is that a series of convulsions, sometimes leading to death, might occur.

Dr. William Fletcher, scion of a well-known Indianapolis family, was appointed superintendent of the Indiana Hospital for the Insane, replacing Dr. Rogers in 1883. Fletcher became famous for burning all the restraints in the hospital on Christmas Day, 1883.

Anna Agnew remembered:

> . . . with amusement the perfect storm of indignation that was aroused among the attendants when soon after Dr. Fletcher's appointment as superintendent, he abolished mechanical restraints of all descriptions. This action of the superintendent, together with the fact of his making a bonfire of the restraints in the presence of the majority of the patients, and accompanied by religious services, singing, prayer, etc., was at the time commented upon in all the [Mid] Western newspapers, very few commending the wholesale sacrifice, many considering (while they did not directly approve of the system of restraints) that the manner of getting clear of the objectionable article, might have been managed with less of the sensational phase.
>
> But the attendants, what a blow at their dignity! What a curtailment of long established fearfully abused power! How they did splut-

ter. "Only think of it. Not allowed to twist arms, can't even 'cami-sole.' Why don't you think, the carpenter came in today and took out the very last one of our restraint chairs. How ever we are to manage the set in our ward, the Lord only knows. And don't you forget it, every single one of the nasty things knew before two days that we did not dare restrain them any more. Oh, its just too bad."

I believe it is generally conceded that the change was a benefi-cial one, both to patients and conscientious attendants. The wards are sweeter—as to atmosphere—and pleasanter to the sight. Since the majority of restraints are suggestive of possible outrages in the hands of irresponsible people, I have frequently heard such remarks as the following from the attendants: "Who is the best judge of the propriety of restraining a patient, the physician who only sees the person for a few moments each day, when of course the patient knows enough to be quiet, or us attendants?"

Knows enough to be quiet!—knows enough always to feel that in a kind and considerate physician they have a friend at court, and it is well indeed not to give this authority into the hands of [atten-dants] who do not know enough to be trusted; to remember that these [patients], so unfortunate as to be obliged to stay there, are human. . . .

I do not entirely disapprove of the use of certain restraints; in-deed, at times, under judicious persons, I consider them a kindness. I know there were nights when it would have been a merciful act to lock me in a crib so that I could not have gotten out. The cribs were simply a bedstead (such as we all used) with a lid over it. But there were a number of those same old cribs that added bloody brilliancy to the historical bonfire.

Camisoles were the notorious straightjackets, strapping patients' arms and hands to their bodies. Restraint chairs were bolted to the floor and the patients strapped in with their wrists in cuffs. When she was restrained in order to prevent a suicide attempt, Anna Agnew did not complain. She saw value for them in such circumstances, unless restraints were used punitively and applied in an abusive way.

British psychiatrists had been more concerned about the use of restraints than their American counterparts. Dr. John Conolly had abolished restraints at the Hanwell Pauper Lunatic Asylum in 1834. Dr. John Charles Bucknill of the Devon County Lunatic Asylum reported in 1853 that the use of mechanical restraint was only justified in a small number of cases. At the annual meeting of the Association of Medical Superintendents of American Institutions for the Insane in 1874 there were long discussions about patient restraint. Dr. Bucknill attended the meeting in 1875, offering a wager to any American superintendent who could find restraints on any wards in British asylums. Apparently there were no takers.

Dr. Fletcher wrote in his annual report:

> *Moral force methods are stronger than physical restraints in aiding the mind to recover its balance. This firm belief has caused a warfare upon chemical [sedatives] and mechanical restraints in the wards of the Hospital to the degree that the use of 209 restraint chairs, 120 cribs, 101 camisoles, 107 restraint straps, 56 wristlets, 55 pairs of gloves, 11 pairs of anklets, and 2 leather collars have been abolished; while yet a few cases are restrained by some of the gentler means, during short periods of their occasional excitement, it is hoped that in a short time, with more skilled help and better prepared rooms, that no vestige of such means shall remain.*

Before leaving as superintendent of the Indiana Hospital for the Insane in 1887, Fletcher encouraged the state legislature to investigate abuses at the hospital. He was not new to politics. He had been elected a state senator in 1882 the year before he became superintendent. The hospital investigating committee issued a thirteen hundred-page report including charges of high payments for shoddy supplies and poor quality food for patients as well as incompetent attendants. The qualifications of the president of the hospital board were questioned.

After leaving the state hospital, Dr. Fletcher established a private psychiatrictreatment facility, "Neuronhurst." His academic duties continued. He was considered by many to be the leading psychiatrist in the city.

Dr. Fletcher was described as humane, and his innovations at the Indiana Hospital for the Insane bear this out. His own experiences as a prisoner might well have made him especially sympathetic to patients confined in a hospital and in restraints.

A lifelong friend, Morris Ross, was quoted in an obituary as writing that Fletcher:

> . . . *had no enemies in the usual sense. He might differ with individuals and tramp on their favorite feelings with the ruthlessness of a boy in a garden, but he so loved humanity that he was hardly sensible of personal enmity. Manifestly an endowment of this sort will find life a more or less thorny thing . . . but this shall have no other effect than to stimulate that rare courage . . . to such natures at all times applies the great truth that much is forgiven because he loved much.*

Fletcher wrote of the mystery of insanity: "There is something sacred about insanity—the traditions of every country agree in throwing a halo of mysterious distinction around the unhappy mortal, stricken with so sad and lonely disease . . . we cannot face the breathing ruin of a noble intellect undismayed. The broken sounds, the vague intensity of that gaze, those whisperings that seem to commune with the world of spirits, the play of those features still impressed with the signet of immortality—though illegible to our eyes, strike us with awe . . . how forcibly must the wreck of mind itself, and the mournful aberration of that faculty by which most we assimilate to our Maker, humble our self-sufficiency."

In addition to this sympathetic view of patients, embellished in typical Victorian language, he was capable of skepticism about some of the theories of his day and wrote in an annual report of the hospital, "In examining the application papers of female patients, a large number, perhaps the majority of them, have the cause of their mental derangement attributed to diseases peculiar to their sex, whether true or not is a question difficult to determine."

Among the honorary pallbearers at his funeral in 1907 were the poet James Whitcomb Riley and Senator David Turpie. Mrs. Fletcher had died in 1904. Six of their children remained. Although he had established Neuronhurst, he had no stock in it and left his family no fortune, his estate being estimated as less than ten thousand dollars. A colleague described him as "caring for money only as a means to perfection and of culture."

Anna Agnew met the new superintendent in an unusual encounter, typical of Dr. Fletcher:

On Sunday morning of June seventh, 1883, while the attendants were preparing the patients for their usual walk, and I, together with several other old clods, was waiting to be taken across the hall into another ward to stay until their return, the back door very near "my corner" opened, and a gentleman came in alone, walking up to me, he said pleasantly, "How do you do this morning?"

I had not the most remote idea whom he was, neither would it have made the slightest difference if I had known. He had offered me his hand, and, of course, was simply mocking my well-known delusion. Every body, I thought, knew that my hand was accursed, so roughly turning away, I said, "Oh you go to hell," my favorite place of consignment.

He looked at me just for an instant as though utterly confounded and said, "Go where?" in a perfectly exasperating tone; then pausing a moment said, "No, indeed, I won't go there; I don't believe I should like that climate. And now then," he continued, "wouldn't you like to go out riding or walking this lovely morning?" and I said,

"No."

Then he said, "What's the matter with you anyway? Do you know what you do want?" And I, growing more angry every moment, said, "There's nothing at all the matter with me, and I want you to go about your business and let me alone." Then his manner changed, and he said decidedly, "That's exactly what I don't intend to do. It is my business not to let you alone any longer. I understand you have not had your foot upon the ground in two years. Why, that's dreadful. Now then, inside of ten minutes, I will bring my porter, and he and I will pick you up, rocking chair and all and carry you down stairs," and off he went. And this was my introduction to Dr. Fletcher, our new superintendent.

Did he execute his threat? A moment or so after, our supervisoress, a young lady whom I had always liked, came bringing a hat which she began trying on me saying kindly, "Are you going to allow Dr. Fletcher to make such a spectacle of you as that;" And I answered, "Does he think I am a damned fool?" "No," she answered, "he thinks you a very determined, obstinate woman, and you will find him equally determined. Now, do come with me," and giving me her arm, we walked down stairs.

This was the man under whose humane management I remained until well. The proof of which was a discharge to myself, at my own solicitation, "as a person of sound mind, competent to control my own actions and affairs," instead of being discharged to my county, subject to the sheriff's action; in which case I would become either the poor house pauper which my husband intended or be a dependent upon the charity of my relations.

Do not understand that I was immediately restored. My convalescence was slow, and attended by many painful, mortifying scenes, the memory of which even now brings the blush of wounded feeling to my cheek. I was so often, so horribly misunderstood.

William Fletcher

Dr. William Fletcher was accustomed to experiencing, or precipitating, "the sensational phase" as Anna Agnew called it. He had enlisted in the Union army in the Civil War. Another physician was available for the unit so Fletcher volunteered instead for intelligence service, a dangerous duty. Captured in Virginia by the Confederates, he destroyed the notes and maps he had made, lighting his pipe with them as he sat by a campfire. Fletcher was kept in solitary confinement six weeks and made two escape attempts, receiving a bayonet wound. In October 1861 he was tried, court-martialed, and sentenced to death. General Robert E. Lee commuted his death sentence.

While in Libby prison in Richmond, Virginia, he was identified as a physician. Through an administrative error, he was paroled and took charge of a gangrene hospital. Gangrene, a severe wound infection, was a leading cause of death in the Civil War. The only treatment at the time, seventy years before antibiotics, was amputation of the wounded, infected extremity.

Released in an exchange of prisoners brought about by his brother, Miles Fletcher, superintendent of the Indianapolis Public Schools, he returned to Indianapolis and resumed the practice of medicine. He also worked in the war effort with the Sanitary Commission, the Civil War equivalent of the Red Cross. In addition he traveled to several battlefields to provide medical and surgical help to the wounded. Fletcher gave lectures about his experiences in the war and donated the proceeds to providing supplies for soldiers in hospitals. He was sent to Terre Haute, Indiana, to look after the condition of military prisoners there and gave his well-publicized lecture to local citizens as well.

The Fletchers were a prominent Indianapolis family. Calvin Fletcher, William's father, had moved from Vermont to Ohio, where he taught school to support himself while studying law. He arrived penniless in Indianapolis in 1821 just a few years after Indiana had become a state. In addition to arguing some well-known legal cases, he began to invest in land quite successfully. He became a banker and civic leader and was famous locally for a diary covering his life from Vermont to just before his death in Indianapolis in 1866.

William Fletcher's education had begun at a new log schoolhouse in Indianapolis and continued later at the county seminary. He studied at Asbury (now DePauw) University in Indiana. In 1855 he prepared for entrance to Harvard but elected instead to work for Louis Agassiz, learning zoology and botany from the famous scientist and Harvard professor. His ability at sketching and making clay models undoubtedly helped in these studies. He began medical studies at the College of Physicians and Surgeons in New York City in 1856, graduating in 1859. Following graduation, he practiced medicine in Indianapolis until entering military service.

After the Civil War, Fletcher traveled in Europe for a couple of years, studying at hospitals in Paris, London, Glasgow, and Dublin. Subsequently, he practiced medicine in Indianapolis and helped to establish the Indiana Medical College in 1869, at one time or another holding chairs in physiology, anatomy, material medica (pharmacology), practice and therapeutics, and, eventually, nervous and mental diseases.

In 1870 he established the Indianapolis City Dispensary, a clinic for the poor and for prisoners in the jails. He later held the Chair of Nervous Diseases at the Central College of Physicians and Surgeons of Indiana, one of the schools that were eventually to come together as the School of Medicine of Indiana University.

There were many more medical colleges in late-nineteenth-century America than is the case today. At the turn of the century, proprietary medical schools were combining with universities. This led to a much better level of medical education than in the nineteenth century.

Dr. William Fletcher was superintendent of the Indiana Hospital for the Insane from 1883 to 1887. He had married Agnes O'Brien of Boston, a nurse whom he had met while she was working in a hospital in New York when he was a medical student. Anna Agnew mentioned Mrs. Fletcher favorably as being much concerned with helping patients and as doing her a kindness in spite of rude remarks Anna made when she was quite depressed. She thought Mrs. Fletcher the loveliest character she ever imagined.

Anna Agnew also wrote of the kindness of another physician at Seven Steeples, Dr. Thomas:

> Probably the perusal of extracts from letters written to my sister and others during my early convalescence, all of which were preserved and returned to me after my complete recovery, will better explain my peculiar state of mind than any thing I now say. All women know the luxury of tears, as well as men misunderstand them. But for five years not a tear came to relieve my sorrow or moisten my burning eyes. And to my dying hour I will remember when they came thick and fast with choking sobs—and what a blessed relief they were too.
>
> All from a kind voice saying, "Mrs. Agnew, is there any thing I can do to make your sad surroundings pleasanter; and will you promise not to hesitate to ask me for any favor within my power to grant?" I could not answer for tears. Call this childish weakness, if you please. I was more helpless than a child, in my loss of self-control, and I had so long been unused to kindness [from Dr. Walker and Madame C.]. Dr. Thomas, the kind considerate friend referred to, deserves the confidence of all having the welfare of the afflicted at heart, and he has the affectionate regard of all his patients.
>
> My sister having been in constant correspondence with Dr. Thomas, wrote to me by his advice, saying so many letters had been sent me without a word of reply, but that she felt now that surely I would send her a line and that she would write at length. . . . But I had gotten so completely unaccustomed to writing, that I felt but little inclination to reply to her letter until in answer to the doctor's question, "are you going to write to your sister?"
>
> I said, "No!" And he answered, "Now! I am disappointed in you! If you could read the number of good letters I have read from that good sister about you, certainly you would send her, if no more, a line to relieve her of long waiting, and I have assured her you would write."

Anna Agnew had actually written a lengthy letter to Dr. Thomas before this time, explaining some incidents on the ward and attempting to clarify the position of kindly attendants about whom she feared he had been misinformed. She also discussed with him her delusions about the Masons and some of her concerns about religion: "I tell you, Dr. Thomas, you are probing deeper than any mortal knows." This suggests that he was reading her writings as part of what would now be called journaling and employing methods that were precursors of present-day psychotherapy.

Dr. Fletcher encouraged her to write letters about her experiences to an Indianapolis newspaper to which he was a contributor and might well have encouraged her to write her book. Drs. Everts, Hester, Rogers, Thomas, and Fletcher wrote testimonial letters, published at the end of the book.

Dr. Fletcher started a school for patients, many of whom were illiterate. Those who were adept at sewing and other crafts displayed their products in the reception room, thus being complimented and appreciated, Anna Agnew thought. Proceeds from sales went to the hospital treasury. Musical instruments, books, and pictures were provided on the ward for a homelike appearance.

One building was used for several purposes, including as an amusement hall:

> I remember well the night it was dedicated, as Dr. Fletcher said to fun, crowded with employees, of which in the different departments there are several hundred, he called upon them to pledge him their support in his efforts to ameliorate as far as possible the gloom of the unfortunates under his charge, and right noble they responded, with cheer after cheer, for Dr. Fletcher as he, leading his wife out upon the floor, opened the ball playfully compelling her to go through the quadrille [in] spite of her protestations that she could not dance.

Dr. Fletcher instituted another innovation for the Indiana Hospital for the Insane. In his Annual Report for 1883 he had recommended that a female physician be appointed for the Department of Women. In 1884 he noted, "In my last report I suggested the appointment of a female physician for the Department of Women, and shortly afterwards nominated Dr. Sarah Stockton for that position. I am pleased to report that results have shown the wisdom of that appointment in the general and special improved condition of the female patients under her charge. She has had to take charge of one division of the house [the Department of Women] as a general practitioner, and do all the special work for the whole establishment, and has given complete satisfaction in every capacity."

Dr. Sarah Stockton was a pioneer in an America where women were generally excluded from mainstream medical education. She was one of only a few hundred women practicing medicine in the United States at the time and the first to practice at the Indiana Hospital for the Insane. She was one of twenty-two women physicians working in eighteen state hospitals in nine states.

Sarah Stockton had been born in 1842 on a farm near Lafayette, Indiana, and later operated the Stockton House hotel in Lafayette with her sister. She graduated from the Women's Medical College of Pennsylvania in Philadelphia in 1882 and returned to Indianapolis to practice medicine in a private practice and at the hospital for the insane. Dr. Stockton served on the State Board of Charities, which oversaw state institutions, and at one time was physician in charge at the Indiana Women's Prison in Indianapolis. For twenty-five years, until her death in 1924, she served full-time as a physician at Central State Hospital. Anna Agnew wrote:

> I don't think my sisters of the woman's rights party will care to claim me as one of them. Indeed I doubt very much if I understand what they really wish in the matter of rights any better than the majority of them do themselves. I've had a sufficiency of female

sufferage! [*sic*] And not having any property need not concern myself about the justice or injustice of taxation without representation,
or make any exertion to understand the difference between misrep-
resentation and taxation. There now! I'm all mixed up! Won't some
of my learned sisters straighten me out?

I won't venture a single idea upon civil or uncivil service or the
tariff but upon one reform—of woman—I do with all my soul sanc-
tion her education as a physician! And for the sake and in behalf of
suffering woman—insane women in particular—since they can not
tell their misery, I make an appeal to the board of trustees of every
female hospital for the insane in the land, for the appointment of a
woman upon their medical staff.

I often tell my dear friend, Dr. Stockton, that I still think her a
handsome woman! But I felt the first time she came into my darkened room, where I lay in such agony as only miserable women suffer, and seating herself at my bedside, looking pityingly at me, the
expression in her lovely blue eyes in itself a mute promise of assistance, before a word was spoken, that an angel had been with me.

Am I too enthusiastic? If I could only express the hopefulness her
words inspired, not that I cared then to live, for I did not, but I was
so thankful to be relieved from my terrible physical sufferings, and
she was so handsomely dressed, too! And such lovely diamonds! And
as I had a woman's admiration for lovely things and only a child's
self control, I immediately began appropriating her rings which she
seemed not to notice. So, for a few brief moments, I was the happy
possessor of life-long, coveted diamonds!

And I still retain my admiration for my friend, and have added
to my admiration of her personal appearance and intellectual en-
dowments—love—for her never failing kindness and sympathy toward me in my sorrowful life. Thus this advantage one possesses in
having a woman for your physician. If you love her you can tell her
so. In the other sex you must tell his wife how much you think of
her husband, and that's a satisfaction, too, when you also love the
wife since there's not that woman lives who does not like to hear

nice things said of her husband. It is indirectly a delicate compliment to her good taste since she chose him or was chosen by him.

Anna Agnew seemed ambivalent about some aspects of the women's movement; perhaps it was just the same independence she had expressed about religious denominations and the current belief in spiritualism. During the period from the 1870s to after the turn of the century women, especially the wealthy, had gained some property rights, but overt legal discrimination still existed. Susan B. Anthony was jailed for trying to vote in the 1870s. In the centennial year 1876, she proposed a Declaration of Rights for Women. It was not recognized officially, however, at the celebration in Philadelphia honoring the Declaration of Independence of 1776.

In the pre-Freudian era in which Anna Agnew was writing, her reference to love for Dr. Stockton probably reflected flowery Victorian expression more than what would later be called "transference." She might also have been mildly manic while writing this passage. ["There now! I'm all mixed up!"] Dr. Stockton's approach to her appears professional and kindly in the context of the time and of Anna Agnew's illness and not part of what would currently raise concerns about interpersonal boundary issues in the doctor-patient relationship.

In addition to his other reforms, Dr. Fletcher employed a precursor to recreation therapy in twentieth-century psychiatric hospitals and encountered some of the same difficulties recreation therapists do today when psychiatric inpatients are taken to community activities:

The last summer I spent at the asylum I attended a circus. Forepaugh [Circus] was in Indianapolis, and Dr. Fletcher arranged for a circus party that, I am sure, has no precedent in any other asylum. I was entirely well but was invited to go with the party, consisting of twelve insane women, Dr. Fletcher, our gentlemanly druggist, and four attendants, besides myself, started in town, three miles distant, to attend the evening exhibition. Reserved seats had been provided, and all went smoothly; one old German lady, as we reached the ground, seemed in danger of becoming separated from the crowd, and our "drug store man" [hospital pharmacist] as she called him went to help her along when she cried out so as to attract attention, "Shtop now, Got in himmel! Shust you look after some old beobles, and let young beobles pe, I shust dinks Dr. Fletcher pe pretty vell known here, and if I gets lost, I say I shust be one of his kinder, by golly!" She was over seventy years of age.

Very soon we were quietly seated, and the doctor remarked that he did not think his crowd presented any thing of an unusual appearance, any more than many other crowds of the same size; they were all nice looking and quiet.

I said, "but, Doctor, suppose it was announced in this quiet tent that one dozen lunatics from the asylum were here in a crowd, don't you imagine there would be more reserved seats vacated suddenly than would be filled again tonight?" and he said, "How would it do to have a jolly good performance of our own after the regular programme is gone through?" and he had not long to wait before our own performance began.

I think the doctor must have supplied himself liberally with small change before he started, but I imagine several bills also were exchanged before the scenes closed. Our crowd completely monopolized the ice cold lemonade, popcorn, and candy stock, but the fun reached the screaming point when the peanut man began calling out his delicious wares, "Here's your fresh roasted peanuts just out of the hopper." Now my uninitiated friend you are not obliged to laugh since you don't understand the significance of the "hopper" in hospital parlance [the place where soiled linens were deposited] you might not have considered it so excruciatingly funny as we did.

When one of our party sang out, "Just out of the hopper, well I'll be damned! Go to hell with your damned old peanuts just out of the hopper!" and when Dr. Fletcher, pressing his arm around her, said, "You be still, Laura," she, "That's all right, doctor, give me another squeeze, it's been a devilish long time since I've had a man's arm around me!" I am sure no one in that circus party will ever forget that night, and I think the doctor was fully convinced of the ability of his crowd in the way of performance, independent of programme or precedents, so my readers will understand that gloom does not universally prevail among the insane.

Other recreational activities broadened the experience of patients under Fletcher. When Anna was recovering near the end of her hospitalization, she played the piano for other patients to sing: "Oft in the Stilly Night" and "Then You'll Remember Me," and others of the "dear old songs, sweeter and purer than any of the new ones, until a feeling almost of peace came to my troubled heart." On one occasion she provided especially memorable entertainment for her fellow patients:

> And not only was my music a comfort to me, it was also entertainment for the unfortunates around me, and many a curious concert we held, as one and another would call for some favorite song or hymn, as an encouragement to me in my efforts to pick out a suitable accompaniment, that they would help me sing. Once I remember "Aunt Betty" saying, "Do sing 'When I Can Read My Title Clear to Mansions in the Skies;' and I said, "But I didn't read my title clear, Aunt Betty," and she answered, "Well do sing it anyway, for I do thank the Lord!" and as I began singing, and several others joined me in the chorus, "We will stand in the storm, and we'll anchor bye-and-bye," she began shaking hands with others gathered around and crying, "Glory! Glory!" in regular Methodist camp-

meeting style, until the excitement became contagious, as all religious excitements do, and one young girl, an excellent elocutionist, mounted a table and began an exhortation, partly in fun and partly in earnest; another one turned down several chairs in a sort of circle around the piano improvising a mourner's bench, and began calling sinners to come forward and be prayed for, and through it all rang the choir screaming out "We will stand the storm," and storm it was, and such a revival of religion was inaugurated on the old fourth ward, as to require quite a force of the authorities to quell it. And who dares say there was not quite as much religion in that revival as many similar manifestations outside the bars, and no more levity than is expressed by some of the pious utterance of so-called religious evangelists of the present day. When the doctor heard of it, he said gravely, "Did you start all that hub-bub last night? I'm surprised at you!"

Reform of Psychiatric Institutions

Reform movements in mental health care in America have been cy-
clical. During the first, beginning in the two decades before 1850, the
most well known figure in the crusade was Dorothea Dix. In addition
to writing and teaching children in church classes, she taught school
and established her own school in Boston. In 1841 while teaching Sunday school at a county correctional house in Massachusetts, Dix visited
the inmates. The institution provided detention for defendants await-
ing trial, inebriates, debtors, "idiots," and "lunatics." This experience
was her introduction to the condition of prisoners and the institution-
alized insane. While providing education and religious instruction at
the prison, Dix read about moral treatment for the first time. She toured
jails and almshouses in Massachusetts. A Boston newspaper published
a sensational article by a colleague revealing the conditions she had
observed. Mincing no words, Dix later proclaimed, "I tell what I have
seen. . . the present state of insane persons confined . . . in cages, clos-
ets, cellars, stalls, pens! Chained, naked, beaten with rods, lashed into
obedience!"

Thus began her career of examining state institutions around the
country and lobbying state legislatures for reform of existing conditions.
During this period, state legislatures had begun to view favorably the
spending of some tax monies for public institutions. Actively promoting moral treatment, Dix instigated enactment of laws to develop asylums in fourteen states resulting in the founding of twenty-two new
institutions.

Her fervor in the promotion of asylum building gave her a prominent position in shaping public policy. Finally, she approached the
United States Congress. A senator sympathetic to her cause presented
her memorial to the assembled body in June 1848. Having visited institutions in all but three of the then existing states, she had outlined her
findings including statistical data and proposed federal land grants for

asylums similar to those for institutions of higher education. Unfortunately, the proposed bill finally died in committee, but Congress did establish a Government Hospital for the Insane that served as an asylum for the District of Columbia.

Dix continued her visits to institutions in individual states and ultimately extended her crusades to Europe. She died in 1887 at the age of eighty-five. The previous year Anna Agnew, like many other former mental patients at various times during the century, had published her assessment of the breakdown of moral therapy in overcrowded, understaffed institutions.

The second reform movement, which occurred in the first two decades of the twentieth century, coincided with the publication of *A Mind That Found Itself* by an articulate and well-educated former asylum patient, Clifford Beers. Consistent with the progressive spirit of the times, the mental hygiene movement that Beers helped to found optimistically and idealistically hoped that through healthful living habits mental illness could be prevented. At this time the new developments in psychology and sociology provided hope for thorough understanding of the human mind and prevention and treatment of all psychological and social problems as well as of psychiatric disorders. Unfortunately, psychiatric disorders could neither be prevented nor treated at the time.

Initial optimism faded. The broad perspective that "mental health" could readily be provided for the entire population had been too optimistic.

The third period began in the 1960s and marked the first real change in psychiatric treatment. At last, effective measures to modify the course of psychiatric disorders had become available with the discovery of antidepressants, antipsychotics, and medications to stabilize abnormal mood swings. Social factors played a role as well. Antiauthoritarian attitudes of the 1960s, the increasing role of the government in providing health care, and groups advocating the involvement of patients in decisions about their own care helped to open the door to improved treatment.

As in the rest of medicine, treatment was increasingly outpatient, and hospitalization less frequent. In psychiatry these changes led to the greatest change in two centuries: "deinstitutionalization" and the near demise of asylums. Outpatient treatment in both the public and private sectors and community-based programs became the major loci of treatment.

Reform in the management of health care delivery and expenditures began in the mid-1980s. Management of health care systems and efforts to provide cost-effective treatment used computer programs and other sophisticated technology. "Bottom lines" became important, because costs had risen dramatically. Within a few years "managed care" became "managed cost." That change raised concerns about the *quality* of care that are being addressed now in the twenty-first century.

CHAPTER SEVEN

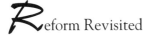eform Revisited

Asylums are no longer the major locale of treatment. Ironically, contemporary methods of cost control in medicine mimic some of the ways asylum superintendents used to fit their programs into limited funds from state taxes. "Fixed budgets, prospective payments, outpatient alternatives, and case management have been driven by the discipline of limited budgets," as psychiratrist Jeffrey Geller has written. In the best of situations patients can be easily moved from inpatient to residential facilities to outpatient care as the need arises. All too often the provision of "all the care needed but no more" is logistically difficult. The system does not constitute a seamless web.

The private sector is now seeing the problems that have long beset public systems. Geller observed: "Many say the public sector is disappearing. That's true only if you define the service system by the payer source. If you define the service system by procedures, personnel, and technologies, then the private sector is disappearing. The public-sector service system has emerged as state of the art. We should give it the respect it deserves and learn from its past errant ways."

No one seems satisfied with our current system of health care in the United States, but proposed remedies vary widely. Health care is an enormous industry. A variety of insurance companies, hospital organizations, citizens groups, professional groups, small businesses, large corporations, labor unions, and others with various agendas and solutions employ lobbyists in Congress and state legislatures. Both the major political parties have allegiances to "special interests." Perhaps the tragic events of September 11, 2001, and emphasis on the need for medical and psychiatric care in emergencies will provide an impetus for change in health care delivery, generally.

What has been the experience in other industrialized countries where many other types of health payment plans exist? A *Wall Street Journal Report* presented data about this question: One method is tax-based systems. In the United Kingdom and Canada health care is controlled by national ministries that regulate every aspect of medicine. Generally, these are the least expensive systems, but the less money a country devotes to health care, the more it limits access. The United Kingdom spends the lowest percentage of gross domestic product (GDP) of any country on health care, 6.7 percent, but patients might wait as long as six months for heart surgery or even longer for non-critical care like orthopedic surgery. Canadians pay higher taxes for more coverage, 9.5 percent of GDP.

A second method of meeting health care costs is social insurance, the system in France and Germany. Quasi-public insurance carriers manage health care. Government regulates these not-for-profit carriers in almost every aspect of their business. The costs are higher than in tax-based systems—9.6 percent of GDP in France and 10.6 percent in Germany—but often provide a high level of care unthinkable in other systems. Insurers are not trying to turn a profit so there is not as much pressure to cut costs. Doctors are not paid as much as they are in the United States. Overhead is lower than in the United States, where it has been estimated that one-quarter of health-care workers do nothing but paperwork.

The third system, the most expensive, is the private insurance system, which is seen in Switzerland (10.6 percent of GDP) and the United States (13.6 percent of GDP). The United States provides the largest and most expensive example of payment for health care. For those who have adequate insurance or other resources, access is impressive. The U.S. currently has the most advanced medical technology, the best-trained physicians, and unparalleled treatment. However, those with less comprehensive coverage or no insurance receive much lower levels of care than individuals in other developed countries with tax-based or, especially, social insurance plans.

In the care of psychiatric patients, cost concerns are not the only problem. Stigma, as well as cost, limits access. Tragically, even in the twenty-first century, the public and patients both still frequently see mental illness as disgraceful and self-inflicted. A recent study in the *American Journal of Psychiatry* by Jo Anne Sirey and her colleagues found that perceived stigma contributed to treatment discontinuation in older adult outpatients with major depressive disorder. Younger patients reported perceiving more stigma than did older patients, but were less likely than older patients to discontinue treatment as a result of stigma.

Psychologist Otto Wahl conducted a survey in the 1990s of a nonrandom sample of nearly fourteen hundred psychiatric patients and former patients recruited through the National Alliance for the Mentally Ill (NAMI). Sixty-one percent of the respondents in Wahl's survey reported that they had at least sometimes been shunned or avoided by others when it was revealed that they were mental health consumers. Like Anna Agnew, they were often rejected by some of their relatives. Some described how others refused to believe that their illnesses were "real," thinking rather that they were issues of motivation, effort, or will—or even a pretense. Interpretations of mental illness as religious failure, spiritual weakness, or sin were encountered. In contrast, 83 percent reported positive experiences of understanding or support at least sometimes and 47 percent experienced these attitudes often. Again, like Anna Agnew, they found some who were sympathetic to their plight.

Although Wahl's respondents did not emphasize physical abuse, that tragedy is still with us. From Clifford Beers onwards writers of memoirs about treatment in the twentieth century have reported abusive practices. In October 1998 the *Hartford* (Connecticut)

Courant ran a series of five articles about 142 deaths nationwide in the previous decade that occurred after patients had been in restraint. The database was formulated from records of public agencies, advocacy offices, and news accounts of deaths in psychiatric hospitals, psychiatric wards of general hospitals, group homes, residential facilities, and mental retardation facilities. These articles were written 115 years after Dr. Fletcher burned the restraints at the Indiana Hospital for the Insane.

While noting that death occurring during restraint is not necessarily caused by the restraint, the *Courant* indicated that many deaths had occurred after restraints were inappropriately applied and not in accordance with acceptable procedure or that patients were left unattended for hours, also against current regulations. Just as Anna Agnew had, reporters realized that <u>attendants</u> have a difficult and dangerous job, yet are often poorly trained and supervised. They also agreed that, appropriately used, restraints can protect patients from self-harm.

Many of the reforms Anna Agnew proposed have been enacted. Medical organizations and institutions and governmental regulatory agencies formulated specific rules aimed at preventing abuses. Routine inspections by authorities had been carried out at the facilities where the deaths reported by the *Hartford Courant* occurred. Although regulations require that only physicians order restraints and that staff must frequently monitor their use, these measures were not always carried out. Cover-ups still occur. Governments sometimes protect their institutions and professionals, their colleagues. Malpractice lawsuits add to concerns about disclosure of abuse.

Only three states were reported by the *Courant* as licensing aides in psychiatric facilities. There is still no uniform, minimum training for psychiatric aides, and they are still poorly paid. Anna Agnew had written more than a century earlier that there would be no remedy for abuse "until state laws require that none but those who are fitted for the sacred duties of attendants upon the insane be employed."

The *Courant* reports noted that fiscal pressures had led to cutting staffing and reducing training required for staff. In addition, as managed care limits access to hospitals, patients seem to be entering the system in more troubled conditions than ever before, putting them at greater risk for being unable to resist abuses.

As in Anna Agnew's day, there can be a disparity between the ideal situation and reality. Similarly, there are efforts to abolish abuse, now as there were then. The 1998 *Hartford Courant* articles discussed progressive methods some facilities are using to do away with most use of restraints. Many individual hospitals and some state and local governments have enforced more thorough examination of the use of restraints, promoted leadership that changes staff attitudes, and implemented training of staff in appropriate methods of dealing with patients. When needed, restraints can be applied briefly, humanely, and with careful monitoring. As Dr. Fletcher had found, the need for restraint can be eliminated in many cases, safely and without exorbitant cost.

CHAPTER EIGHT

*A*nna Agnew after the Asylum

The Keyts in Moscow maintained contact with relatives in Cincinnati. Anna seems to have identified with the well-educated, socially prominent Cincinnati branch of the family. In a letter written after her hospitalization she wrote:

> I used very much to enjoy a visit to Cincinnati, but I spent a month there recently, and really was quite surprised to find so little of the city in town, the greater part having moved out on the hills, Walnut Hills in particular, celebrated just now as being the residence of both the ex and elect Governor of Ohio, and especially being noted as the fountain head of the recent great medical discovery, "Toast and Ale," a sovereign remedy for malaria, typhoid fever and numerous other 'ale-ments' that poor mortals are subject to. Now I stopped there several weeks, in a physician's house, too; and I tried my utmost to get up some sort of miserable feeling, headache, or something of the kind, and hinted very strongly of the efficacy of the prevailing tonic; but not a drop of ale or smell of toast could I get, probably from the fact of the Methodist Conference being in session on Walnut Hills at the time.
>
> Everybody, and their "uncles and aunts and cousins" were going to see the "Battle of Sedan" and certainly the painting deserves the praise the thousands of visitors gave it. I saw it both by day and night, and could see it again with interest.
>
> During my stay there, crowded houses were sobbing with sympa-

thy over "Miss Multon's" woes, as portrayed by Clara Morris' splendidly realistic acting, and crying and laughing over "Rip Van Winkle" and "Schneider." I wonder if I am altogether singular in this respect. I never could induce myself or be induced to weep over stage pictured woe.

Before he had married Anna's mother, Nathan Keyt had been married to Mary Thrasher, a collateral descendant of the Penn family of Pennsylvania and of one of the early families of Maryland. As was all too common at the time, she died a young woman. Dr. Alonzo Thrasher Keyt, Nathan and Mary's only child, became a prominent cardiologist in Cincinnati. Alonzo Keyt held a faculty position at the University of Cincinnati School of Medicine as well as conducting a private medical practice. His research, innovative in its time, delineated some of the diseases of the heart valves and was well known even among cardiologists in Europe.

Anna Agnew admired her half-brother, Dr. Alonzo Keyt, who, like her father, contributed to her intellectual interests. When she was young, he had found her reading his medical books and said that she could have been a doctor were she not a woman. Later when she wrote to him from Indianapolis about Dr. Sarah Stockton, he encouraged the idea of women in medicine. One of Alonzo Keyt's daughters married his associate in medical practice. They had a daughter who, like her father and grandfather, became a prominent physician in Cincinnati. Early in her career she worked at the state psychiatric hospital in Columbus, Ohio.

Dr. Alonzo Keyt had died while Anna Agnew was in the hospital, as she noted in the book. During her visit to Cincinnati after her hospitalization she likely stayed with the family of Alonzo Keyt's son or that of his son-in-law. Both men were physicians. The Walnut Hills area that she mentioned was at the time a fashionable suburb of Cincinnati.

Although many women of lesser means worked in factories, there were not many ways middle-class women could earn money "respectably" at the time. Nineteenth- century authors of reform literature often sold their own publications to readers. Anna Agnew published her book with the firm of Robert Clarke and Company in Cincinnati.

In the middle to late nineteenth century, Cincinnati was the major city for book publishing west of the Allegheny Mountains. The railroads would change that, making Chicago the publishing center for the Midwest, but not before *From under the Cloud* was published in 1886.

Like many other publishing houses of the time, Clarke was also a bookseller. It maintained a London office and imported English and other European books. Clarke might well have been a source of books Anna had read. She later listed her occupation as "book agent" and "canvasser," possibly selling other publications of Robert Clarke and Company as well as her own book. She did not want to become financially dependent on her family.

Anna Agnew's life was changing; Moscow, Ohio, was changing, too. After she visited in 1885, she wrote:

> Dear old Moscow! Older than Cincinnati, the Paris of America. For many years the place and people seemed enjoying a Rip Van Winkle sleep—looking on many things considered modern improvements with suspicious eye—as innovations not to be tolerated by the old families—but gradually these old-timers were obliged to succumb to young blood and ideas and in consequence, now presents quite a looking-up appearance, notwithstanding there are many visible marks of what the Ohio River is capable of doing when on an annual high. It is a lovely, innocent looking stream now, too low for enterprising steamboat men to admire, but to me dear beyond words, in its associations with my happy childhood. On its banks came memories thick and fast, of merry moonlight boat rides, of voices mingling with laughter and song, many of them silenced forever, and all scattered, probably never to meet again.

Anna corresponded with and was visited by her favorite sister and brother-in-law, Lida and George Irwin, while in the hospital and went to live with them after her discharge and her divorce from David. In the early 1870s, George and Lida Keyt Irwin had moved to Pittsburgh, where George worked in a company owned by his uncle James.

James Irwin and Company, manufacturing chemists, had been established in 1840. It was one of the first chemical works in the country, supplying the important glass, iron, and other industries in Pittsburgh. In the late nineteenth century the company was reported in a publication about local industry to "have achieved an enviable reputation for the purity, strength, and excellence of their product and command the best class of trade. Their works are fitted up with all modern appliances, and the most approved processes of distillation and refining have been introduced, under the superintendence of Mr. George W. Irwin and his partners."

The Irwins employed two servants. They were living in fashionable East Pittsburgh, and George Irwin was moving up in the management of James Irwin and Company.

Anna described her life in Pittsburgh in glowing terms:

> While I am writing I am seated before a lovely porcelain-lined, brightly burning grate filled in with natural looking lumps of simulated coal through which glimmers, or glows, or rushes, as 'Old Probabilities' suggests to the thermometer, natural gas, making certainly an ideal fire. Think of it! Down in the basement roars the furnace. Out in the kitchen glows the range. In the dining room faintly gleams the tiny flame only waiting the call of the bell (by simply turning a knob) to spring into brightness. Up stairs into the sleeping rooms through the halls goes creeping the delicious warmth filling the whole house with comfort. All this by the magic of this wonderful gas. Is it any wonder, under its influence, we are prone to forget how treacherous is its nature and workings—how it steals noiselessly out of the slightest imperfection of pipe or fixtures, into

our neighbor's cellar, without the odor of the manufactured article to betray its presence, only waiting the thoughtless appearance of lamp or match to give fearful sign of its presence. So while we enjoy the luxury, we must also take the risk, since there's no rose without its thorn. . . .

But our kitchens here are simply perfection. Indeed, I think our kitchen just now the most desirable place in the house, pleasant alike to mistress and maid. I haven't seen a frown on our Katie's face in a month, and small wonder, since, as she said this morning: "Indade, ma'am, with not havin' to be after liftin' the nasty ashes, nor breakin' me back with carryin' up the coal, sure me work is but play just. And it's meself that's glad of the natural gas." And I said: " So am I, Katie; and in return for all the comfort it affords us, we will give it all the care its dangerous character calls for."

Anna's illness, bipolar disorder, was characteristically episodic. She mentioned having days of gloom and days of extreme gaiety in childhood. The early years of her marriage were characterized by a remission when she felt well and happy. Even after more than seven years of severe depression and occasional mania, she recovered in the absence of any effective treatments. She remained well, except for occasional mildly depressed days, for almost a decade after her discharge from the Indiana Hospital for the Insane.

Tragically, her illness returned. She had another episode requiring hospitalization, this time at the Western Pennsylvania Hospital for the Insane at Dixmont near Pittsburgh. She was admitted on January 5, 1894. George Irwin took her to the hospital and provided the admitting information. Fortunately for Anna, Dixmont, like the Indiana Hospital for the Insane, had a woman physician on staff. Pennsylvania law had required that a woman physician be in charge of care for women patients in state hospitals. During part of the time she was in the hospital Dixmont had a nurses' training school. In view of her plea in the book for trained nurses to care for the insane, Anna Agnew would have approved.

Anna Agnew died at Dixmont Hospital; on March 25, 1917, at the age of eighty. By this time, her beloved sister Lida was gone, and George Irwin had remarried and moved to New York as president of the General Chemical Company of Pennsylvania (successor to James Irwin and Company). He had died in 1913. In hospital records giving the date of her death, Anna is listed as a private patient. Perhaps George Irwin had seen to it that her care was provided for. One of his and Lida's daughters was married and living in Pittsburgh and might have been involved in helping her Aunt Anna.

Anna Keyt Agnew's life had spanned American history from the presidency of Andrew Jackson to that of Woodrow Wilson. Three years after her death women would vote for the first time in national elections, a right Anna Agnew never enjoyed in spite of her interest in politics. As demonstrated by her physician grandniece in Cincinnati, professions became more open to admitting women. Eventually more progressive divorce and custody laws would provide relief from some of the sorrows Anna Agnew experienced. Psychiatric treatment later included family and marriage counseling that might have provided happier circumstances for David and Anna Agnew and their young sons.

Her illness, untreatable and misunderstood during her lifetime, and contemporary laws and customs had cost her a marriage, her children, years of suffering, and loss of belief in traditional religion. Her book bears testimony to her ability to cope with terrible tragedies and daily suffering. We can only imagine that Anna retained her remarkable courage to the end.

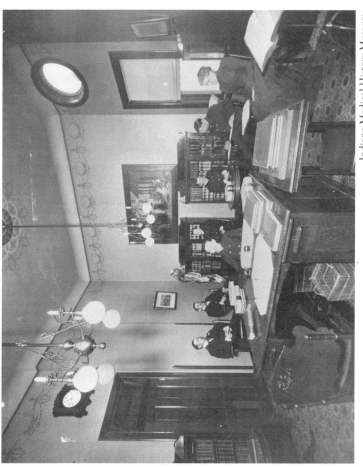

Dr. Sarah Stockton (1842-1924) is seated at right with her colleagues in the physicians' library at the Indiana Hospital for the Insane. Dr. Stockton's thesis for her M.D. degree from Women's Medical College of Pennsylvania, Philadelphia, in 1882 had been on the topic of "Insanity." Dr. William Fletcher appointed her the first female physician at the hospital and wrote that "results have shown the wisdom of that appointment." Her first visit to her patient, Anna Agnew, on the hospital ward left Anna with the feeling "that an angel had been with me."

Dr. William B. Fletcher (1837-1907), who was accustomed to the "sensational phase," burned all the restraints at Indiana Hospital for the Insane in 1883. The conflagration was witnessed by Anna Agnew.

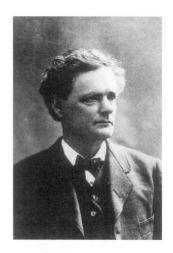

Dr. George F. Edenharter (1857-1923) built a laboratory in the 1890s for the scientific study of psychiatric disorders, the second in the United States. The Pathology Building now houses the Indiana Medical History Museum.

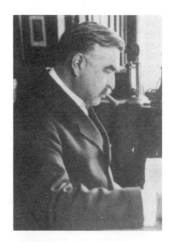

Dr. Max Bahr (1872-1953) studied psychiatry in Germany. He lectured to professionals and the public about psychiatry and encouraged the research of Dr. Walter Bruetsch.

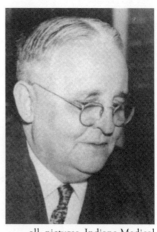

all pictures, Indiana Medical
History Museum

PART TWO

CHAPTER NINE

$\mathcal{S}$olving Anna Agnew's Quandary: The Development
of Psychiatry

The history of psychiatry in the first half of the twentieth century is mirrored in the work of two superintendents at the old Seven
Steeples where Anna Agnew had been a patient. Dr. George F.
Edenharter and Dr. Max Bahr emphasized patient care, teaching,
and research—the cornerstones of present-day medical schools—
from the turn of the century on. Their tenures, thirty years each,
lasted from the 1890s to the 1950s and brought inevitable change.

The association of Anna Agnew's physician Dr. William Fletcher
with medical schools that would train Edenharter and Bahr was
characteristic of changes in medical education in the United States
in the late nineteenth century. In 1869 Dr. Fletcher participated in
organizing the Indiana Medical College; he held chairs in several
departments, including nervous and mental diseases. He later held
the Chair of Nervous Diseases at the Central College of Physicians
and Surgeons of Indiana. These medical schools were involved in
mergers that formed the Indiana University School of Medicine in
the first decade of the new century.

Prior to the 1870s medical schools in this country had been primarily those run by a few physicians in return for fees from students.
Length and quality of study varied widely. Lectures to large classes
with little hands-on laboratory experience were common. Practical experience with patients other than in demonstrations to classes

or observation of doctors in hospitals and clinics was unusual. Many physicians still apprenticed themselves to practitioners.

Physician and historian Kenneth Ludmerer discussed the recommended changes that included longer periods of study, better preparation, more academic training, new courses in science, and higher standards of practice. Returning from study in Europe in the 1870s, physicians such as William Fletcher emphasized the need for scientific medicine.

In the late nineteenth century new or enlarged teaching hospitals opened in Boston, Baltimore, New York, Philadelphia, and Ann Arbor, Michigan. The "Flexner Report" in 1910, which excoriated schools that had been dilatory in employing reforms, was seminal in extending these reforms to all medical schools in the United States. Abraham Flexner, an educator who had visited medical schools around the country under the aegis of the Carnegie Foundation, had prepared the report.

Medical education in the United States began to emphasize laboratory instruction followed by clinical experience in teaching hospitals. Ludmerer observed the climate of reform in the Progressive Era, generous funding for university medical schools and hospitals provided by the new American philanthropists, and innovations in education devised by professors trained in Europe led to a unique system.

Like many of the doctors who were at the institution when Anna Agnew was a patient, Edenharter, the first superintendent in the twentieth century, had had other careers than medicine. Born in Ohio, he moved to Indianapolis in the late 1870s when he was twenty. He worked at the cigar-making trade for about six years. Edenharter was also active in politics and was elected to the city council in 1884 and in 1886.

He had begun the study of medicine as an apprentice to a local physician, and then attended the Indiana Medical College from 1884 to 1886. After graduation he practiced with his former mentor until 1890, when the board of aldermen unanimously appointed him as superintendent of the City Hospital. His administrative skill led to his being chosen in 1893 as superintendent of the Central Indiana Hospital, the new name of the Indiana Hospital for the Insane.

In 1896 the hospital dedicated a Pathology Building that Edenharter had planned and built, creatively using the modest funds available. It utilized the most modern techniques devised in Europe during this period of exciting discoveries in laboratory medicine. In the United States, this hospital was second only to the New York State Psychiatric Hospital in New York City in providing a state-of-the-art laboratory to study psychiatric disorders with anatomical pathology, light microscopy, bacteriology, and blood chemistry. By the time of his death in 1923, the Indiana University School of Medicine had been in operation for almost two decades. The Pathology Building was the location of teaching and research in psychiatry at the school until midcentury.

Anna Agnew would have been heartened by Edenharter's proposal in the 1894 annual report, "We fully appreciate the needs of a [training school for attendants]. Considerable time and thought have been given to the perfection of plans for its organization. A graded course of instruction will be presented by a competent corps of professional men together with the physicians of the institution. Attendance upon the lectures and recitations will be obligatory."

After Edenharter's death in 1923, Max Bahr, a staff psychiatrist at the hospital, became superintendent. An Indianapolis native, Bahr graduated from the Central Indiana College of Physicians and Surgeons in 1896. For a year thereafter he was a physician in the Indianapolis Dispensary established in 1870 by Dr. William Fletcher. He moved for a year to Washington, D.C., where he was chief resident physician at the Government Emergency Hospital. In Washington, Bahr came in frequent contact with the mentally ill patients at the Government Hospital for the Insane and became interested in psychiatry.

Bahr returned to Indianapolis and "with much enthusiasm and

curiosity, I received an appointment on the staff of the Central Hospital on March 1, 1898. At that time the science of psychiatry was almost unexplored territory. The treatment of the insane was merely custodial—housing them, feeding them, treating them kindly. Very little effort was made to cure mental diseases because no one knew anything about them."

After taking a one year leave of absence to study at the University of Berlin, Bahr received the Doctor of Psychological Medicine Degree in 1908. Because of his knowledge of German, he was permitted to study with Professor Theodore Ziehen and translated much of Professor Ziehen's psychiatry textbook into English. In Europe, Bahr would have become familiar with the latest findings of laboratory and psychological research.

Max Bahr was the first physician at the Indianapolis hospital to be trained as a psychiatrist. Specialty training was increasingly a part of the education of American physicians. After World War I even excellent training in four years of medical school was seen as insufficient preparation for medical practice. A year of hospital training after medical school became standard. Additional "residency" training in hospitals and clinics was beginning for those who wished to specialize.

From early in his career Bahr was on the faculty of the new Indiana University School of Medicine, which reported in its 1908 catalog: "The Indiana University School of Medicine is one of the few institutions in the country giving a full practical course in Clinical Psychiatry. The Board of Trustees and Superintendent [Edenharter] of the Central Indiana Hospital for the Insane have erected one of the finest clinic halls and laboratories in the country, and the students of this school are enabled to avail themselves of the clinical facilities afforded only by such an institution."

In 1938 Central State Hospital was described in a national report as having:

one of the largest and best equipped neuropathological laboratories in the country for research in mental diseases. It is closely affiliated with the University Hospitals of Indiana University, and serves as a teaching center in psychiatry for Indiana University School of Medicine. The superintendent [Bahr] is professor of psychiatry and head of the department of nervous and mental diseases of the Medical School, and the director of laboratories [Walter Bruetsch] is clinical professor of psychiatry. There is a training program for residents in psychiatry.

As part of his teaching and clinical work at the hospital, Bahr pioneered everything from psychoanalytically oriented psychotherapy to chemically or electrically induced convulsive therapies. Most important, he and his colleagues performed follow-up studies of patients receiving new treatments to see what worked.

He began social service and occupational therapy teaching and clinical programs and lectures to law students about legal issues in psychiatry. Bahr gave lectures on a wide variety of topics to lay groups as well as to the medical profession. Until mid-century his Saturday afternoon clinical demonstrations to medical students were a cornerstone of education at Indiana's only medical school.

Contemporary with Bahr's retirement and death in the early 1950s, the Institute of Psychiatric Research and a state hospital with clinical research facilities, Larue Carter Hospital, were built on the campus of the Indiana University School of Medicine. Central State Hospital, located two miles distant, became a treatment center for chronically mentally ill patients but maintained some contact with university programs. It was closed in 1994.

Central, of course, to the advance of competent and effective psychiatric medicine is accurate diagnosis of the diseases to be treated. Diagnosis in medicine, the keystone of treatment, has paralleled concepts in Western philosophy going back to the ancient Greeks. Hippocrates, the founder of Western medicine, focused on individual symptoms in individual patients. Other physicians over the centuries assumed that there are disease entities, or groups of symptoms, manifested by similar symptoms in different groups of patients.

In the eighteenth and early nineteenth centuries, psychiatric illness was assessed in *cross-section*, at a single point in time, and interpreted as a response to life events. In the late nineteenth and early twentieth centuries, the development of the anatomical/clinical view of disease led to describing diseases in terms of the correlation of diseased organs or tissues with groups of symptoms that patients experienced and the *longitudinal* course of these symptoms over time.

Dr. Walter Bruetsch at Central State Hospital in Indianapolis worked with other leaders in American psychiatry on the committee that prepared the first edition of the American Psychiatric Association *Diagnostic and Statistical Manual of Mental Disorders*, in 1952. Originally trained as a neuropathologist, Bruetsch worked with the committee categorizing disorders related to underlying disease like infections or tumors of the brain.

As the twentieth century progressed, "explanations in medicine would involve infectious agents, nutritional factors, abnormalities in the immune system, and inherited abnormalities of body chemistry." Philosopher Paul Thagard observed that modern medicine assumes that most human diseases are multifactorial, that is that there are many inherited and environmental factors involved in causing a given disease. This is thought to be true in psychiatry as well.

Vague diagnostic entities in psychiatry early in the nineteenth century contributed to another problem that involved not only diagnostic categories but also procedures for involuntary commitment to asylums. There was concern in the mid–nineteenth century, as there would be in the mid–twentieth century, that individuals with no mental illness were being involuntarily committed to asylums. Two cases in Illinois focused on this issue.

Elizabeth Packard had been committed to the state asylum in Jacksonville, Illinois, in 1860 under contemporary Illinois law that permitted husbands to have their wives committed on the signature of the state asylum superintendent without prior legal proceedings. It is possible to speculate, based on material in family diaries and other resources researched by Barbara Sapinsley, that Elizabeth Packard did suffer episodes of psychiatric illness, perhaps mania. It also possible to speculate, on the basis of her husband's reported behavior and his writing, that he suffered much more severe and prolonged disorders than she, probably severe major depressive disorder as well as, possibly, obsessive-compulsive disorder. Nonetheless, prevailing laws at the time permitted *him* to have *her* involuntarily committed to the asylum. Elizabeth Packard mounted a vigorous campaign in several states to change commitment laws.

Resulting reforms affected the more famous case of Mary Todd Lincoln, widow of the president, later committed by her son Robert Todd Lincoln to a private psychiatric hospital in Illinois. Many historians have described Mary Todd Lincoln's severe depressions as well as possibly manic mood swings. Involuntary commitment of Elizabeth Packard or Mary Todd Lincoln under present-day law would be much less likely than it was in their day. Illness alone is not sufficient cause for involuntary commitment. Patients are involuntarily committed only after a court hearing and only if imminently suicidal or homicidal or severely deficient in the ability to care for their own basic needs.

Superintendents of asylums for the insane were most distressed by these cases because some of them were implicated, especially in Elizabeth Packard's case, in unprofessional behavior. Noted Philadelphia superintendent Thomas Kirkbride wrote in 1880, "In many sections of this country, of late years, a studied effort has been made by a limited number of writers, to create a belief, that sane persons are often confined in hospitals, as insane, by their relations or others, from motives other than to secure their treatment." He explained that "salaries [of physicians] are in no way regulated by the number under their care, and the fewer they have to look after, the less work they have to perform. . . . These institutions would, of all places, be the very best in which to secure the prompt detection of the attempted wrong."

Statistics for diagnoses at the Indiana Hospital for the Insane the year Anna Agnew was committed indicate that asylum physicians recognized that nine patients were "not insane" and discharged them. Data for the year of her discharge indicated thirteen such patients. In some instances at least, individuals who had no symptoms of mental illness were recognized as such and discharged by the hospital physicians. Refinement of diagnoses and more enlightened involuntary commitment laws and procedures makes the possibility of improper commitment much less likely today.

Beginning in the late nineteenth century and throughout most of the twentieth century there was a dichotomous grouping in psychiatric diagnosis between organic and functional disorders. Organic disorders such as delirium and dementia were characterized by deterioration of memory and intellectual function and were related to underlying medical illness and observable brain pathology like tumors and infections. Functional disorders were seen as somehow related to abnormalities in brain function. Nineteenth century physicians realized that disorders in function might represent brain abnormalities that could not be discovered by laboratory techniques available at the time. In the early to mid–twentieth century many practitioners inferred that functional meant that the causes were psychological only.

Among the functional disorders, the term "psychosis" replaced "madness" or "insanity," as Anna Agnew and her physicians called it, and was more narrowly defined as including delusions, hallucinations, and disorganization of thought and behavior. Neuroses, in contrast to psychoses, lacked hallucinations, delusions, and bizarre behavior and were characterized by prominent anxiety. The term, "neurosis," has been used extremely broadly to include almost any mental content or behavior seen as abnormal as well as many specific disorders.

Emil Kraepelin, a German psychiatrist at the turn of the twentieth century, employed accurate description of groups of symptoms and longitudinal studies of patients in his research. He observed hundreds of patients, in a hospital not unlike those in which Anna Agnew had been treated, and followed their cases for years. His research led to the differentiation of two of the functional disorders: dementia praecox (schizophrenia), a chronic thought disorder, and manic-depressive psychosis, an episodic disorder of mood. Most patients with mood disorders have depressions only (major depressive disorder). Some, like Anna Agnew, experience both manias and depressions (bipolar disorder). Predicted outcomes do not occur in every case. There is some overlap between categories. Diagnostic categories do not completely fulfill the ideal of discrete entities.

Reminiscent of some of the conflicts around the situations of Elizabeth Packard and Mary Todd Lincoln, concerns about the meaning of diagnosis and its relationship to commitment to psychiatric hospitals resurfaced in the 1960s. Deconstructionist theories in philosophy and history were applied to medicine and psychiatry as well. For example, Michel Foucault's *Histoire de la folie* in France and in R. D. Laing's *The Divided Self* in England examined the ways physicians had devised constructs of disease .

Well-known and, to say the least, controversial books in the United States included Thomas Szasz's *The Myth of Mental Illness* and Erving Goffman's *Asylums*. It was postulated that there is no such entity as mental illness and that all psychiatric treatments tend to be repressive and demeaning to patients, benefiting only the practitioners. Because carefully defined and studied diagnoses were not yet in widespread use in America, and asylum practices were still not always ideal, their concerns had a basis in fact as well as in philosophy.

Until 1980 psychiatric diagnosis in many locales in the United States was reminiscent of theories of disease in the early nineteenth century. In a study seen as a scandalous exposé in the early 1970s, David Rosenhan arranged for eight normal individuals to pose as patients and to seek psychiatric hospital admission on different occasions to twelve hospitals in five states. Their only complaints were hearing voices that said, "empty," "hollow," or "thud." No symptoms, including the complaint of hearing voices, were simulated after admission. These pseudopatients were hospitalized from seven to fifty-two days, nineteen days on average. No staff detected their status, but some of the other patients did. Many were diagnosed schizophrenia. Rosenhan saw these findings as proof that diagnoses have no meaning. No classification system from Kraepelin onward, however, would have indicated that his pseudopatients met diagnostic criteria for schizophrenia or anything else. Use of the diagnostic systems adopted by the American Psychiatric Association in 1980 would have prevented this travesty.

In the current American *Diagnostic and Statistical Manual of Mental Disorders* the old organic versus functional dichotomy is no longer used. The former organic disorders are now designated as delirium, dementia, amnestic (memory), and cognitive (intellectual) disorders. They are still characterized by deterioration of memory and intellectual function and are related to underlying medical illness. Research in recent decades has demonstrated that functional frequently means abnormalities in the function of chemical messengers in brain, the neurotransmitters, the action of which is influenced by both inherited and environmental factors.

"Psychosis" is still the term used for disorders such as schizophrenia that are characterized by hallucinations, delusions, and bizarre behavior. Diagnoses formerly included under neuroses have been more carefully defined, and the term, neurosis, is no longer used officially.

Why bother with refining diagnoses? Simply put, we now have effective treatments. If a psychiatrist does not know what major depressive disorder, bipolar disorder, and schizophrenia are, he or she will not know which patients would benefit from the use of antidepressants, mood stabilizers, or antipsychotics. If family, social, economic, and other problems in a patient's life are not assessed, it is not possible to employ effectively marital, job, family, or other counseling or psychotherapy, and any benefits of medication are dissipated by the consequences of personal and social problems. In the case of delirium, dementia, amnestic, and cognitive disorders it is crucial to diagnose the underlying medical/surgical condition and to treat it appropriately.

One of the interesting correlations with psychiatric illness is that bipolar disorder seems often to be associated with creativity. Anna Agnew and others who wrote nineteenth-century asylum reform literature suffered from this disorder. It had long been thought that there is a relationship of "madness" to the artistic temperament. But it is not just any madness; we now know that it is specifically bipolar disorder.

Data from many studies one presented in *Eminent Creativity, Everyday Creativity, and Health* demonstrating that individuals with mood disorders are more likely than others to engage in creative pursuits. It has been suggested by Ruth Richards that the relatively high lifetime prevalence of mood disorders in the population (1.6 percent for mania and 14.7 percent for depression in the population studies of psychiatric epidemiologist Ronald C. Kessler and his group) is related to the natural selection of those with the positive trait of creativity which seems related to intervals between severe extremes of mania and depression. Anna Agnew wrote her book when she had recovered.

The present level of understanding of disease in psychiatry necessitates establishing correlations of a variety of factors with specific disorders in order to elucidate their causes. Because the current psychiatric diagnostic system is descriptive, any diagnosis can be the focus of research into correlated factors whether they be genetic, neurochemical, neurophysiological, psychodynamic, psychological, social, or anything else. Diagnostic criteria can be modified when new research data are available. Treatments can be studied for efficacy and used successfully even if causes are not fully understood.

Biological and psychological, like nature and nurture, are no longer meaningful dichotomies as they were thought to be in the early to mid–twentieth century. Nobel laureate Eric Kandel, a psychiatrist as well as a laboratory scientist, has contributed to contemporary understanding of the age-old mind/body problem.

Kandel has hypothesized five principles. First, "all mental processes . . . derive from operations of the brain." Second, genes and the chemical reactions under their control are important determinants of the functions of brain cells and the connections between cells. Thus genes exert significant control over behavior, which is a result of brain cell activity.

Third, "social and developmental factors" as well as genes are necessary to explain either normal behavior or a given mental illness. Fourth, changes in genetically controlled chemical reactions in the brain, induced by environmental factors, contribute to the biological basis of individuality and presumably are responsible for initiating and maintaining psychiatric disorders. In other words, what happens in the environment affects brain chemistry and the chemical reactions genes control. "All of 'nurture' is ultimately expressed as 'nature.'"

Finally, psychotherapy or counseling becomes effective when it produces long-term changes in behavior, presumably doing so by altering genetically controlled chemical reactions in the brain. Heredity and environment are inextricably intertwined, not separate entities opposed to one another.

In the last half of the nineteenth century, the promise of discovery of causes and cures for specific diseases had come with the development of laboratory science, especially the study of infectious diseases. Such discoveries seemed no longer a matter of speculation but, rather, amenable to the scientific methods developed by Pasteur in France, Koch in Germany, and others.

Advances in light microscopy, the discovery of specific tissue-staining techniques, and the ability to grow bacteria in laboratory cultures outside the body made study of the infectious diseases possible. Bacteria could now be seen under the microscope using dyes specific to particular types of bacteria to make them stand out in a magnified tissue section, and they could be grown in the laboratory

Meanwhile, the use of penicillin begun during World War II made the more drastic and less effective fever therapy obsolete. Bruetsch was one of the psychiatrists chosen to study the new medication. In the 1940s he described the culmination of a quarter century of his research devoted to treating paresis, "penicillin, if given in sufficient amounts, is superior to malaria therapy. I would not be surprised if this study means the end of the malaria treatment, which has never been an ideal way of treating [paresis], but which was the best possible means of benefiting this otherwise incurable brain disease."

In the first half of the twentieth century psychiatry was not usually so fortunate in the development of new treatments. Given the absence of specific medication or other treatment for most psychiatric disorders, new knowledge in medicine and surgery was adapted to psychiatry, often unsuccessfully. Enthusiasm for scientific medicine led to some even more drastic treatments than malarial fevers.

Egas Moniz, a neurologist in Lisbon, and his colleagues performed the first prefrontal lobotomy in 1935 by severing neural tracts connecting part of the frontal lobes to the rest of the brain. It was hoped that this treatment might help the chronic, severely disabling disorder schizophrenia for which there was no treatment. Some severely chronically ill "back ward" patients in state psychiatric hospitals did benefit. About one third of those treated were able to leave the hospital, but they were not likely to resume completely normal function. Patients with mood disorders, especially major depressive disorder, seemed to benefit more than those with schizophrenia. But the surgical treatment was necessarily invasive and resulted in personality changes.

Prefrontal lobotomy was used rarely for the treatment of severe obsessive-compulsive disorder. By the 1980s, it was known by that the nerves that had been severed by lobotomy produce the neurotransmitter serotonin, now understood to be important in major depressive disorder as well as in obsessive-compulsive disorder and a number of other psychiatric disorders. Newer drugs, such as Prozac, also affect serotonin and also benefit patients with major depressive disorder, obsessive-compulsive disorder, and certain other disorders without the personality changes produced by lobotomy.

Convulsive therapies which were also developed in the 1930s, utilized knowledge from neurological and medical discoveries. The reasons for thinking they would be effective, like the hypotheses about chloral hydrate in Anna Agnew's day, were incorrect. There was hope that these treatments would alleviate schizophrenia, but again it was depression and mania that seemed most likely to benefit from induced convulsions.

Initially, convulsions were induced by the hormone insulin which lowers blood sugar, or by pentylenetetrazol, a drug that not only causes convulsions but also decreases the amount of oxygen in the brain. In 1938 Ugo Cerletti and Lucio Bini in Italy introduced electroconvulsive therapy. Electrically induced convulsions are much safer than insulin or pentylenetetrazol induced seizures because the treatment is much briefer and does not decrease the amounts of oxygen or blood sugar, the major nutrients of the brain. Paul Huston and his colleagues at the University of Iowa demonstrated in the 1940s that the new electroconvulsive treatment shortened from twenty-one months to fifteen months, on average, an episode of major depressive disorder. As a result patients' hospital stays were shortened and their suffering diminished.

Convulsions produced by small amounts of electrical current applied to the temples (now provided by high technology equipment that monitors electrocardiograms and electroencephalograms simultaneously), administered after brief intravenous anesthesia and muscle relaxation, remain the most effective treatment for episodes of major depressive disorder. Such treatment would have benefited Anna Agnew's depressions and manias and shortened her hospital stays. In most patients today, however, medications alleviate episodes of mood disorder. Electroconvulsive treatment is used only for those severe and refractory depressions in which current medication/psychotherapy regimens are of little help.

ample, elegant techniques for electrical recording of brain activity and noninvasive brain imaging of intravenously injected radioactively labeled chemicals, all computerized, are making it possible to begin to understand what abnormal chemical reactions are associated with the various psychiatric disorders and how particular medications alter them.

All of this comes down to the study of chemical messengers in the brain: the neurotransmitters. Individual nerve cells, or neurons, including the billion or so in the brain, produce and transmit electrical current. They work as does a very complex computer through millions of connections among the cells in the various parts of the brain. But the ultramicroscopic gap (synapse) between cells is not bridged by an electrical spark. Rather, when a neuron fires, a neurotransmitter is released onto receptors on the next neuron in line to make it transmit the electrical current. More than a hundred brain chemicals are thought to act as neurotransmitters.

Neurotransmitters such serotonin, norepinephrine, and acetylcholine had been identified in nerves in the body during the first decades of the twentieth century. They had been identified in various parts of the brain by midcentury, but their role there was less than certain. It turns out that multiple chemical reactions form neurotransmitters in brain cells. When the neurotransmitters are sent out by one cell to connect with other cells, they start chains of chemical reactions in other cells in order to maintain the electrical activity of the brain. Various steps in these chains of chemical reactions are important in psychiatric disorders and the medications that treat them. Chemical reactions are under the control of multiple genes, whose action is modified by the internal and external environment.

Studies of brain chemistry at the molecular level have made it possible to begin to understand how neurotransmitters and medications attach to neurons and affect their functions. Computer simulations of the structure of molecules and their chemical reactions hold out the possibility of devising new drugs without guesswork.

Computers have replaced the descendents of Dr. Cade's guinea pigs.

The early twentieth century saw psychologically minded psychiatrists beginning to take over a field that had previously been primarily the province of superintendents of asylums for the insane. This change is reflected in the name of the American Medico-Psychological Association, successor to the Association of Medical Superintendents of American Institutions for the Insane and predecessor to the American Psychiatric Association. In contrast to treatments used in asylums that dealt with large numbers of severely ill patients, psychotherapeutic techniques were more likely to be used with individual outpatients who were less severely ill.

In late-nineteenth-century Europe, trends in thinking about man were interwoven with ideas in developing psychological science in three ways: renewed interest in aspects of the mind that are not conscious to explain behavior that might seem irrational; studies of how the environment is perceived and how that perception influences decisions and behavior; and efforts to understand behavior by observing it without delving into questions of what was going on inside the mind. Sigmund Freud and his followers were concerned with the unconscious. Wilhelm Wündt and the German experimental school of psychology focused on the perception of the form, or gestält, of the total environment. Ivan Pavlov in Russia studied conditioned reflexes and learned behaviors. Later, in the twentieth century, concepts of existential philosophy were incorporated into psychotherapy.

The original psychoanalysts in Freud's school assumed that all feelings and behavior are related to mental content that is not conscious. In order to live life to the fullest and to utilize his capacities to the utmost, an individual must develop insight into many of the unconscious drives and conflicts. Psychiatric symptoms were seen as the result of striving among the unconscious drives or motives and the various psychological defenses of the individual against the behavioral expression of these drives. Freud's method of therapy was to have the patient lie on a couch where he could not see the therapist and to free-associate about anything that came to mind.

Carl G. Jung and Alfred Adler were in Freud's original group in Vienna but broke away early in the twentieth century to found their own schools of psychology. Jung recognized the importance of anthropology, culture, and spiritual values in the development of the individual. He, like many others since, saw psychotherapy as a conversation with patient and therapist face-to-face. Alfred Adler focused on social influences. Adler originated child guidance clinics, group therapy, and family therapy.

Wilhelm Wündt, whose work influenced Kraepelin, developed the German experimental psychological tradition before the turn of the twentieth century. Wündt and his successors studied how we perceive and interpret the environment. The environment, they postulated, is perceived as a whole, rather than as a collection of individual parts. As we perceive it, the whole of the environment is greater than the sum of its parts. Understanding the perceptions of a person helps to understand his behavior. Why he does what he does is related to how he perceives the environment around him rather than to unconscious drives.

Between the two world wars many of these theories were reflected in the work of psychotherapists who began to expand classical Freudian psychoanalytic theories to include more emphasis on cultural, social, and anthropological factors in the development of normal and abnormal personalities. Harry Stack Sullivan in the United States saw interpersonal interactions as important in the development of an individual. The environment helped to shape an individual, as he was involved with others. Ego psychology placed increasing emphasis on the behavior of the individual in current life situations. Object relations theory emphasized positive and negative internal representations of self and other.

In the late nineteenth century in Russia, Pavlov began to study classical conditioned reflexes in dogs. In his classic experiment a dog that normally salivates when food is presented is given food while a metronome ticks. After a number of trials, if the metronome ticks even when no food is presented, the dog salivates. The dog has been conditioned to salivate when a metronome ticks.

Later B.F. Skinner in the United States developed methods for the operant conditioning of spontaneous behaviors rather than automatic reflexes like salivating. For example, a monkey might gradually be taught to put tokens into a machine to obtain peanuts. Trial by trial, only behaviors closer and closer to the machine and then closer to the token slot in the machine are rewarded by peanuts. Finally the monkey receives peanuts only when tokens are put into the slot. Behavioral psychotherapists use these kinds of paradigms to help patients change inappropriate behaviors.

Many therapists objected to an emphasis entirely on observed behavior, although they recognized the value of behavioral techniques. Thus they combined a focus on behavior with attention to the patient's cognitions, or perceptions, that led to that behavior. They attempted to change both behavior and the individual's understanding of his or her behavior. Cognitive-behavioral therapy encouraged patients to outline carefully their unrealistic beliefs about a variety of situations that were preventing them from behaving productively.

An important trend in all psychotherapies in the twentieth century, based both on clinical experience and on economic realities, has been increasingly brief therapy. From Freud's original psychoanalysis that required one-hour sessions five days a week for several years, psychotherapy has gradually been changed into fewer, sometimes shorter, sessions at less frequent intervals conducted during a briefer time frame. Homework by patients, often utilizing computer-programmed learning, is used. These are sophisticated methods of accomplishing what moral therapy tried to do in having patients examine their unproductive behaviors.

Existentialism includes a wide range of twentieth century philosophies. In the turmoil and tragedies of the century it attempted to give some hope for human existence. Existential psychotherapies have provided ways of helping psychiatric patients to deal with their suffering even though causes and cures might not be understood. Each individual is encouraged to find meaning for himself in his unique situation.

Existential therapies focus on choice and responsibility. For example, the existential psychotherapy of Viktor Frankl, who survived a Nazi concentration camp, points out that even in the unimaginable horror of the death camp a person could find meaning in life and still have some choice remaining. He could behave cruelly toward fellow sufferers or he could treat them with kindness.

The development of these and other psychotherapies in the twentieth century has been influenced by the parallel growth of the social sciences. All of the various types of psychotherapy have been employed in working with couples, families, or groups of many types. These have grown out of many of the concepts discussed above as well as sociological theories about how families and groups function. Practitioners of psychotherapy include psychiatrists, psychologists, social workers, and other counselors from a variety of training backgrounds and theoretical perspectives.

Increasingly, therapists of all perspectives are discussing ways that each therapy contributes to helping patients and are defining common threads that link all the approaches to psychotherapy. Research is being conducted about outcomes of the various therapies, that is, which therapies work best for what patients.

As the variety of treatment options and therapist availability opened up, outpatient venues and treatment in smaller private facilities evolved to parallel treatment in gradually depopulated state institutions. When William Fletcher, Anna Agnew's doctor, left the Indiana Hospital for the Insane, he established a small private hospital, Neuronhurst. Later, in the first half of the twentieth century, Max Bahr would advocate outpatient clinics for follow-up of patients after hospital discharge at the state hospital.

Two books about asylum life in the first half of the twentieth century marked the beginning and end of the asylums' declining years. Clifford Beers had been in an asylum and had recovered from what was probably bipolar disorder. In 1908 he wrote *A Mind That Found Itself*, in which he criticized punitive use of straightjackets and seclusion and the lax supervision of untrained, sometimes brutal, attendants. In 1946 Mary Jane Ward published a novel, *The Snake Pit*, criticizing harsh practices in public mental institutions. It made a hero of an understanding psychiatrist who practiced a combination of psychoanalytically oriented psychotherapy and the intravenous amytal interview. World War II military psychiatrists had used this interview technique to induce memories of traumatic events and provide rapid recovery of soldiers at the front.

Beers's book heralded the beginning of the mental hygiene movement. Established in 1909, the National Committee for Mental Hygiene emphasized outpatient clinics, aftercare following hospitalization, and social work services. It had dark days later when a few of its members, in a misinterpretation of the hereditary components of illness, supported legal regulation of who might marry, restriction of immigration of "undesirables," and involuntary sterilization of the mentally ill and mentally retarded. These very destructive theories and practices died out after the Nazi horrors of the 1940s, as did the positive but very broad emphasis on mental health for all the public rather than on treatment of the mentally ill. The National Mental Health Association, organized in 1979, became an advocate for the mentally ill. Its membership comprises both consumers and professionals.

At the same time that medications for treating psychiatric disorders were developed in the 1950s and 1960s and psychotherapies were shortened in time and broadened in scope, there was public outcry about conditions in large public institutions. All of this was reflected in a variety of governmental policies. The Hill-Burton Act in 1946 contributed to funding for new community hospitals, many of them with psychiatric units. The National Institutes of Health in Bethesda, Maryland, developed research programs in medical science conducted in its laboratories and, through grants, in universities around the country. The National Institute of Mental

Health brought the federal government into active support of psychiatric treatment, education, and research. Research and teaching fellowships and stipends for psychiatry residents were granted in the 1950s and 1960s.

After World War II the influx into the United States of physicians, especially psychiatrists, from around the world provided an important source of professionals to staff the developing programs for psychiatric treatment. International medical graduates who entered the expanding psychiatric residencies have made a major contribution to American psychiatry. The American Psychiatric Association has taken a strong stand against the more recent jingoistic rhetoric seeking to limit the number of physicians immigrating to the United States from other countries.

The Community Mental Health Services Act in 1963 created local mental health boards to develop outpatient psychiatric clinics, inpatient general hospital psychiatric services, and rehabilitation, consultant, and educational services in the community. Unfortunately, as psychiatrist H. Richard Lamb observed, there was conflict between the needs of the severely mentally ill, who were increasingly being discharged from hospitals on newer medications and in need of multiple basic services, and the well-intentioned focus of many staff on psychotherapy and patients with less severe conditions.

In 1965 the federal government established two health benefit plans, Medicare for the elderly and disabled and Medicaid for individuals and families with limited income. Private, usually employer sponsored, health plans also developed rapidly after World War II although some had been in place in earlier decades. In the 1970s and 1980s Congress passed legislation that would further change health care financing. The HMO Act of 1973 permitted health care practitioners to organize Health Maintenance Organizations to compete with private insurance. The Employee Retirement Income Security Act (ERISA) in 1974 encouraged employers to create their own employer-managed health benefit plans.

Throughout this time there was constant controversy stimulated by lay and professional groups alike about establishing parity for psychiatric illness. In other words, health plans should provide benefits for those with mental illnesses equivalent to benefits for medical/surgical conditions. The unfortunate reluctance on the part of insurance and other plans to do so had a historical basis. Prior to 1950 hospital stays in large public psychiatric institutions, although not as long as in Anna Agnew's day, were still on the order of months and sometimes years. Private institutions using psychoanalytic techniques often required long hospitalizations for therapy. Long hospital stays would mean higher costs for insurers.

After the advent of pharmacological treatments, briefer psychotherapies, and emphasis on outpatient treatment, these concerns had much less relevance. Nevertheless, a certain unwillingness to pay for psychiatric treatment, whether with taxes or insurance premiums, continued. This lack of enthusiasm on the part of legislatures and insurers reflected the continuing stigma associated with mental illness as well as the reluctance of many psychiatric patients to come forward to demand services for fear of being identified as "mental" patients, thus compromising employment and other aspects of their lives.

The last half of the twentieth century was an era of dehospitalization. Lamb quoted figures that in 1955 there were over 559,000 patients in state hospitals. By 1997 there were fewer than 62,000 patients in these facilities. During this time the total population of the United States had almost doubled from 150,000,000 to more than 260,000,000.

Geller has reviewed the changes in mental health care in the late twentieth century. In public mental hospitals in the 1950s overcrowding and underfunding continued. Nevertheless, there were also efforts at rehabilitation to prepare patients to develop skills necessary for their return to the community. In the 1960s, state hospitals continued to redefine their roles with an increase in outpatient treatment and further expansion of rehabilitation. Unfortunately, community programs and family resources were not always sufficient to provide all the services that patients would need after hospital discharge.

An important and all too often unrecognized factor after the 1960s was the increasingly widespread availability and use of addicting substances of all kinds. Cocaine, marijuana, heroin, and designer drugs were no longer the province solely of marginal or bohemian groups in society but were easily obtained by anyone. Their use temporarily alleviates the pain of mental illness, but heavy use of these drugs worsens the course of any psychiatric illness and makes medication dangerous and psychotherapy and community services useless. As members of the baby boom generation reached their teens and twenties, when many psychiatric disorders have their onset, a new class of severely, chronically mentally ill patients emerged as emphasized by historian Gerald Grob. Many of them were dependent on addicting drugs.

In the 1970s money and interest moved from state hospitals to the community. Innovative programs reflecting a mirror image of nineteenth century psychiatry developed. Then, almost all treatment was inpatient. A hundred years after Anna Agnew entered the hospital, almost all treatment was outpatient, and much of the inpatient treatment took place in a matter of a few days to a few weeks in private hospitals paid for by insurance. In both private and public sectors, day hospitals, intensive outpatient programs (half-days or evenings several times a week), residential and halfway houses, and other innovations became prominent treatment venues.

Concerns about how much of which treatments were needed by whom continued into the 1980s and were heightened in the 1990s with more sophisticated evaluation of the outcome of treatment. One of the unfortunate effects of the dehospitalization pattern of the 1970s had been an increase in the homeless who were neither utilizing nor being fully served by mental health clinics. Some still need asylum.

In contrast to individual patients writing their hospital memoirs in the nineteenth century, groups of former patients and their families organized in the 1960s and took an increasing part in advocating for change in psychiatric treatment and availability of and payment for treatment as discussed in a review by Phillip R. Beard of the Menninger Clinic. The general reform climate of the 1960s and 1970s contributed to the formation of such groups. Consumer groups confronted the psychiatric establishment with the antipsychiatry philosophies of the time.

Later groups changed the focus of patient advocacy. One of the most important of these was the National Alliance for the Mentally Ill (NAMI) which was formed in 1979 and currently has over 200,000 members. The National Depressive and Manic-Depressive Association focuses specifically on patients with mood disorders. Psychiatrists and neuroscientists work with these groups as well as with the National Mental Health Association. Such organizations espouse consumer responsibility as basic to better service and emphasize that change will only be achieved through vigorous advocacy.

Leona Bachrach, who has researched and written extensively about mental health care, provided a thoughtful review of state mental hospitals at the end of the twentieth century. In her opinion, it is impossible to say how mentally ill individuals will ultimately fare in the twenty-first century because of the profound and rapid changes in managed care.

Bachrach reviewed data on four important questions. First, what is the current view of state mental hospitals and how is it different from that early in the twentieth century? Some state hospitals provide innovative programs for care and rehabilitation and others serve as gateways to integrated services as has always been the case. However, some still attend only to basic survival needs and provide little hope for patients. Meanwhile, media attention to abuses in the latter has put all such facilities under increasing public pressure. There is a concern that we will return to an "either-or" perspective—that state hospitals are always necessary or never necessary—without consideration of marked differences in patient needs and in services provided by different hospitals.

Second, Bachrach asked what patients are currently being served by state hospitals? Short-stay patients now represent the majority of those admitted. They might well have multiple admissions with outpatient care in the interim. Even with modern treatments, some recently admitted patients are so severely and chronically ill as to be unlikely to be discharged, and other patients who have been in the hospital for years are considered poor risks for discharge into community living. Many factors influence a patient's ability to live in the community: diagnosis; severity of illness; level of function; and demographics. In addition to individual patient characteristics, community factors are involved such as local and state laws and regulations, the residential and outpatient services available in a given community, and the willingness of that community to tolerate such patients outside the hospital.

Her third question addresses what has happened to mentally ill persons who are no longer served in state hospitals. Many have been successfully treated in community-based service settings. For them, dehospitalization has worked. Others have been discharged into communities with few if any programs to serve them and live on the streets or are frequently incarcerated in prison systems where little care is available. Even when community care has been thoughtfully conceived and adequately funded, some mentally ill patients receive inadequate treatment. Among other problems for those released into the community is the easy availability of alcohol and addicting drugs. The mentally ill who are not receiving adequate treatment often live in disadvantaged neighborhoods because they cannot function in the workplace to earn rent money and easily become victims of drug dealers who are only too willing to accept their disability or unemployment checks.

Finally, what *is* an appropriate role for state hospitals now? Bachrach notes that trying to answer this too often leads to "geography games." The winner in the state mental health system is any-one who places patients somewhere other than in the state hospi-tal, still widely viewed as "inherently undesirable." Outcome crite-ria include decreases in number of admissions, lower patient cen-suses, and shorter lengths of stay rather than appropriateness of ser-vices, quality of care, and quality of life. It is easier to collect num-bers than to try to evaluate services. The numbers all too often impress the public and legislatures. In summary, dehospitalization has been beneficial for some, not for others. The important point is that we look at which patients need what services and how best to provide them.

Anna Agnew had been hospitalized both at the Indiana Hospi-tal for the Insane in Indianapolis and at Dixmont State Hospital near Pittsburgh in the late nineteenth and early twentieth centu-ries. Dorothea Dix had played a role in the history of both. She had encouraged the Indiana legislature in building the hospital for which funds had been set aside. Not only was she involved with Pennsyl-vania officials in the founding of Dixmont but also, according to her biographer Thomas Brown, she assumed a key role in the ongo-ing affairs of the new hospital in Pennsylvania in the 1850s and provided continued attention to the daily administration. The hos-pital was named for her.

Both asylums where Anna Keyt Agnew was treated have been closed. The Indiana hospital was closed in 1994 under allegations of patient abuse that would not have seemed unusual to Anna Agnew a century earlier. On June 12, 1994, the *Indianapolis Star* reported, "Central State Hospital . . . which opened in 1848 and once housed 2500 patients, is empty now and will shut down com-pletely at the end of the month."

On December 2, 1994, the *Star* reported on the trial of two at-tendants who had been charged with negligence in the drowning death of a patient in a bathtub prior to the closing of the hospital. The patient was said to have had orders for twenty-four hour obser-vation, but attendants were said not to have been present for some time. The attorney for one of the attendants was quoted as saying that they were underpaid, overworked staffers who were not trained to handle such an emergency. The judge agreed to an extent with the defendants' attorneys in saying that the evidence revealed that the hospital failed to provide some workers with adequate training and supervision. The judge was reported to have noted that this did not excuse the defendants of negligence, and they received suspended prison sentences and were to complete two hundred hours of community service.

The Pennsylvania authorities closed the aging, historic buildings at Dixmont in 1984, patient care being provided in other newer facilities elsewhere and through outpatient services. Although located in a rapidly developing area, the property was not sold for some time because of toxic materials in the buildings and grounds. In January 1999 a developer bought it, promising to clean it up according to environmental regulations and to build a residential and retail complex. This did not happen immediately. As 2000 drew to a close, Dixmont was described as a burned-out shell.

CHAPTER TEN

*A*nna Agnew and the Twenty-first Century

Anna Agnew advised that we become concerned about psychiatric illness: "Let the public make this a personal matter, since there is scarcely a family exempt from this fearfully increasing malady." She addressed stigma:

I meet many persons who express surprise that I am not at all sensitive regarding my insane experience, and others who regard me a little doubtfully, as though possibly I may not even yet be exactly level, and others again who are so surprised and so very sure "you know," that nothing of the kind will ever come to them because nothing of that sort ever was in "our family!" . . .

During my early affliction, while yet at home, I felt terribly that probably my children might be taunted by unthinking persons over my condition, and one day when there were no one else present but my two eldest boys I said to the eldest one, "Do they ever say at school that your mamma is crazy?" He gave me a troubled look, but before he could reply the other one . . . sprang up with flashing eyes and clenched fist and said, "Yes, sir, mamma, yes, sir! One boy did say that to Dadie, and Dadie! He just up with a darnick and let him have it right on the head, sir!"

She also observed that stigma was not universal:

Only a very few of the old friends [in Moscow, Ohio] are left, and to those few my homecoming [after hospitalization] was as one from the dead. And yet how gladly they welcomed me, and without the slightest reference that could offend to the shadow that for so many years darkened my life.

She made a plea to family and friends of the mentally ill:

Unfortunately, for all concerned, I was not taken to the asylum for a period of several years after the time when common sense, if not common humanity, should have decided that such was the only proper place for me. Right here let me implore those persons so unfortunate as to have friends needing such restraint, not to cherish the old-timed, ignorant idea of some thing disgraceful being attached to this form of affliction; and above all, keep from the stricken one the shadow of reflection that they have disgraced their family since they are insane. The bitterest, most indignant feelings toward my friends were born of this very thought. I sincerely believe that the miserable record of those years, the impressions made and received by me, when my case was so cruelly, or ignorantly, which? misunderstood outside of the asylum, made seven years inside of its walls a necessity, for which I must hold my immediate family, in a measure, responsible, granting at the same time, they intended kindness to me in keeping me home.

If she were alive today, Anna Agnew would be delighted that treatment is now available to alleviate symptoms of bipolar disorder. She had written, "insanity is becoming every year better understood—and though there may be an inherent tendency in that direction, science and the surroundings may combat if not entirely prevent it." Complete (primary) prevention is not yet possible but the secondary prevention of early recognition and treatment is well within modern capabilities. Long-term, permanent cure is not possible, but symptoms of individual episodes can be cured. Continued pharmacological/psychological regimens, when necessary, can prevent or diminish future episodes.

In the best of all possible current situations, the early phase of her illness might have been recognized in her childhood and treatment begun then by a pediatric psychiatrist. If her illness were not recognized until she was an adult, it would have been identified by a well-trained family physician and appropriate pharmacological treatment instituted. Because she had manias as well as depressions, she would likely be referred to a psychiatrist. If necessary, a few weeks of intensive outpatient care for several hours weekly, or even a brief hospitalization for several days, would be utilized. In the hospital, nurses trained to work with psychiatric patients and trained psychiatric technicians would staff the ward.

The hospital chaplain would have training in psychology. Many churches now sponsor counseling centers for families with problems rather than preaching hell-fire-and-damnation for the "sin" of mental illness or attributing human suffering to "God's will" and therefore intractable. Anna Agnew might well have been able to retain a spiritual faith without giving up appropriate skepticism.

Her level of psychiatric care would be varied depending on the severity of her illness: hospitalization, intensive outpatient programs, and increasingly briefer and less frequent outpatient office visits as she improved. When an episode remitted, identifying possible future symptoms that might necessitate treatment again would be discussed with her. She would be encouraged to seek professional help were she to experience recurrence of the illness or troublesome family and social problems that might contribute to relapse.

At all points professionals involved in her care would educate her and her family about the nature of her illness, its prognosis, and treatments available. Marriage counseling and family therapy, conducted by psychologists, social workers, or other trained therapists, would help her and David and the children through the difficult period of severe illness in a wife and mother. Suicide attempts, administration of medication to her children with resulting charges of homicidal behavior, and divorce and break-up of the family could probably be prevented. Had divorce resulted anyway, enlightened laws about mental illness, divorce, and custody would have made it possible for her to care for her children when recovered or, certainly, to see them.

In decrying a change of administration at the Indiana Hospital for the Insane after false accusations against physicians based solely on political changes in the state government, Anna had made another plea:

> Authorities would find oft times that the testimony of [patients], who are debarred from even a voice in matters of importance, would be invaluable in their interests, and quite, if not more, reliable than those allowed to testify under oath. And in this case had the patients (certainly the most interested parties) been allowed to vote, I'm thinking the verdict would have been different.

In the best of modern facilities she would be involved in treatment planning, as a treatment team of all professionals would meet to work out her treatment plan. Her family, also, with her permission, would be apprised of treatment plans and their concerns addressed.

Instead of having to publish a book on her own and sell copies one by one to the public as she and other nineteenth-century reformers did, she could participate in her local chapter of National Alliance for the Mentally Ill (NAMI), the National Depressive and

Manic-Depressive Association, the National Mental Health Association, or other self-help, educational, and advocacy groups. If she chose to do so (and Anna Agnew probably would!) she could write articles and speak to public gatherings under their auspices. Increasingly sophisticated and sympathetic portrayals of mental illness in the media, promoted by these groups, would have set the stage for family and friends to understand the need for, and availability of, effective treatment.

Both Anna and David Agnew would likely have availed themselves of more education. Both would be working in good, probably professional, jobs. If very lucky, Anna would be in a work situation providing opportunities like childcare in the workplace or various part-time employment options for women with small children. Federal family leave legislation would have helped this family during her illness.

The opening chapters of this book described the ideals of moral treatment. Anna Agnew's book reported what happened when moral treatment broke down in large institutions with insufficient numbers of trained staff. Chapter 9 described the current possibilities in a best-case scenario—the optimum of theory and practice. Chapter 7 indicated some of the realities Anna Agnew might face today. Fragmentation of health care and health care financing in the United States often limits access to medical care. Stigma continues to affect patients with psychiatric disorders.

The *New York Times Magazine* reported that the United States, which has the finest available health care, has been ranked fifty-fourth among nations by the World Health Organization in terms of equality of access to that care. The same publication reported an estimate that on any given day, approximately eighteen million Americans meet the diagnostic criteria for mood disorders and decried the fact that the indigent who are depressed are often overlooked and receive little or no treatment. The article made a case that treatment of poor citizens with diagnosable depression might well make significant inroads into the problems of poverty, an enormous benefit to society to say nothing of alleviating the suffering of individuals.

The surgeon general's report of December 1999 reviewed extensive data about mental health care services. Although almost 30 percent of adults in America have a diagnosable psychiatric disorder, less than one-third receives treatment in one year. Some do not seek care because they believe the disorders will go away. Of the majority who perceive a need for care, many do not seek it. Eighty-three percent of the uninsured and 55 percent of the privately insured who do not seek care worry about potential costs. Even though patients with Medicaid have government benefits to pay for mental health care for the indigent, they do not always receive such care. Almost 60 percent of Medicaid patients list as a concern an inability to obtain an appointment soon enough because of an insufficient supply of services.

In spite of data indicating that the rise in mental health care expenditures in recent years has been about the same as for health care generally, insurance coverage of mental health services is typically less generous than that for general health. Harking back to the institution of tax-supported asylums in the early nineteenth century, the private sector still depends upon the government to play a larger role in financing mental health services compared to overall health care.

Columnist Dan Carpenter of the *Indianapolis Star* noted in April 2001, "a new generation of drugs has given countless mentally ill persons their lives back by profoundly easing their symptoms without the debilitating side effects of older medications. . . .They're a mighty bargain compared to the cost of hospitalization, imprisonment and inability to hold a job." He was concerned about the opposition of some state officials and politicians to allowing these medications to be prescribed for Medicaid patients. Their initial costs would be higher than the older medications although patients are much more likely to follow drug regimens when there are fewer side effects, thus preventing a great deal of costly institutionalization and other costs to society. We can imagine Anna Agnew demonstrating with the Mental Health Association at the statehouse. This time, she would not be alone in her pleas to the legislature.

The surgeon general's report observed further:

> Having health insurance—and the nature of its coverage and administration—are critical determinants of such access. But so are factors such as the person's clinical status and personal and sociocultural factors affecting desire for care; knowledge about mental health services and the effectiveness of current treatments; the level of insurance co-payments, deductibles, and limits; ability to obtain adequate time off from work and other responsibilities to obtain treatment; and the availability of providers in close proximity, as well as the availability of transportation and child care. In addition, because the stigma associated with mental disorders is still a barrier to seeking care, the availability of services organized in ways that reduce stigma—such as employee assistance programs—can provide important gateways to further treatment when necessary.

In 2001 the Institute of Medicine (IOM), which advises the federal government issued a 335-page report from its committee on quality of health care in America. The committee comprises individuals with a wide range of expertise, including clinical and research professionals, business and health policy leaders, executives from a variety of health care settings, and representatives of consumer groups. It spent a great deal of time and reviewed extensive data about health care, references to all of which are documented in the report.

In the executive summary it noted: "What is perhaps most disturbing is the absence of real progress toward restructuring health care systems to address both quality and cost concerns, or toward applying advances in information technology to improve administrative and clinical processes. . . Mergers, acquisitions, and affiliations have been commonplace within health plan, hospital, and physician practice sectors. Yet all this organizational turmoil has resulted in little change in the way health care is delivered. . . . Leaders of health care institutions are under extraordinary pressure, trying on the one hand to strategically position their organizations for the future, and on the other to respond to today's challenges, such as reductions in third-party payments, short-falls in nursing staffing, and growing numbers of uninsured patients seeking uncompensated care."

The committee well recognized the enormity of the change that would be required. Noting that the health care system must focus greater attention on the development of health care processes for the chronic conditions, like major depressive disorder, that afflict many people, they pointed out that about fifteen to twenty-five such conditions account for the majority of health care services.

This committee detailed specific measures to initiate changes in four major areas: 1) the infrastructure that supports the dissemination and application of new clinical knowledge and technologies; 2) the information technology infrastructure, itself; 3) payment policies in health care; and 4) preparation of the health care work force.

It concluded its summary optimistically: "Perfect care may be a long way off, but much better care is within our grasp. The committee envisions a system that uses the best knowledge, that is focused intensely on patients, and that works across health care providers and settings. Taking advantage of new information technologies will be an important catalyst to moving us beyond where we are today."

While not giving all the answers, the report provides a number of specifics about how to start the process of change. In spite of their optimism, committee members did not envision that the complete process would be easily or rapidly accomplished—they were confident that Americans can have a health care system of the quality of care they deserve. The current care systems cannot do the job. Changing systems of care will.

As discussed in earlier chapters of this book, many players and sectors of society are involved, yet there has seldom been an effort to look at the big picture. The report of the Institute of Medicine asks that policymakers, purchasers, regulators, health professionals, health care trustees and management, and consumers commit to a national statement of purpose addressing the health care system as a whole. The aims of the system should be health care that is safe, effective, patient-centered, timely, efficient, and equitable.

Nowhere have both the good and the bad aspects of current medical care in America been more dramatically demonstrated than in the horrific destruction of the World Trade Center, September 11, 2001. Long-term plans for dealing with disaster made it possible for victims to be evacuated to many excellent medical facilities in New York City. At the same time, according to media reports, staffing cuts as a result of managed cost left gaps in the ability to carry out some of those plans at these facilities in a way that health care professionals might have preferred.

Coordination of care across all services for all patients is emphasized in the IOM report, as is the importance of teamwork among professionals. As discussed in the best-case scenario for Anna Agnew in the twenty-first century, teamwork has long been a part of the best facilities for psychiatric care, possibly because so many different types of skills are needed to provide for all the needs of psychiatric patients.

Previous chapters in this book have discussed advances in medical education. The IOM report emphasized the importance of using newer technologies to provide information to health care workers about the latest findings of research and how to apply those to clinical outcomes.

The report noted that although payment is not the only factor that influences provider and patient behavior, it is an important one. It suggests that payment methods should: provide fair payment for good care; provide the appropriate information for consumers and purchasers to evaluate differences in health care so that they can make informed choices about where to seek and pay for care; tie financial incentives to the best possible practice of medicine and the achievement of better patient outcomes rather than simply to cost savings; reduce fragmentation of care; and establish pilot programs to test ways of doing this.

In other words all members of the health care system should get their acts together and coordinate services. Part of the change in the system would involve monitoring of all these processes and correcting problems that arise.

In outlining ways to begin such a massive overhaul, the committee pointed out that we now invest annually $1.1 trillion, or 13.5 percent of the nation's GDP, in the health care sector. Estimates indicate that the figure will be more than $2 trillion by 2007. The committee suggested a commitment on the order of $1 billion (a fraction of 1 percent of current expenditures on health care) over three to five years to help initiate the transition to new forms of care delivery. In the long run, beginning to fix the system will be far less expensive than continuing the current system.

The surgeon general reported in the introduction to his December 1999 report that promoting adequate mental health care for all Americans who need it will require, "a societal resolve that we will make the needed investment. The investment does not call for massive budgets; rather, it calls for the willingness of each of us to educate ourselves and others about mental health and mental illness, and thus to confront the attitudes, fear, and misunderstanding that remain as barriers before us."

These reports focus on the need for resolve on the part of each and all of us, as citizens, to work for needed changes in the health care system. Nearly everyone, at some time or another, needs health care. Nearly one-third of us, at some time or another, need mental health care. The responsibility for change ultimately rests with all of us.

In the final paragraphs of her book, Anna Agnew described the debate she had with herself and others about whether or not to publish the book. In the twenty-first century she would be involved in the debate about how best to provide health care, especially mental health care, in the United States. We must make decisions, not easy and not simple, about this issue. The final words of her book apply to our dilemma:

"What is the verdict?"

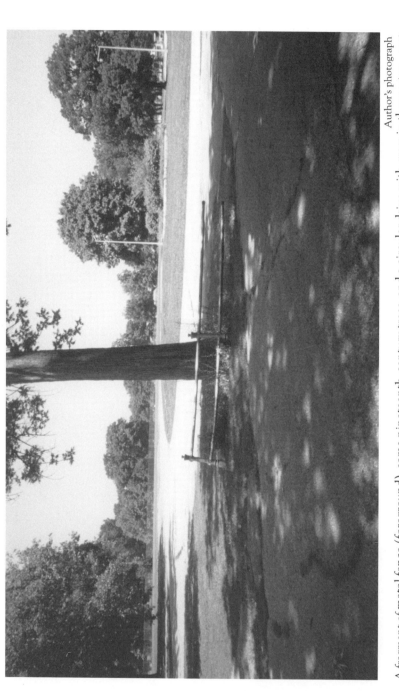

Author's photograph

A fragment of metal fence (foreground), some nineteenth-century trees, and a circular drive with grass in the center—not flowers and a statue—are all that remains of the Women's Building (Seven Steeples) where Anna Agnew spent years at Indiana Hospital for the Insane.

SELECT BIBLIOGRAPHY

Nancy C. Andreasen, "Creativity and Mental Illness: Prevalence Rates in Writers and Their First-Degree Relatives," *American Journal of Psychiatry*, 144(1995):1288–92.

Leona L. Bachrach, "The State of the State Mental Hospital in 1996," *Psychiatric Services*, 47(1996):1071–78.

Max A. Bahr, "A Hundred Years of Psychiatry in Indiana," *Journal of the Indiana State Medical Association*, 42(1949):118–24.

_____and Walter L. Bruetsch, "Two Years' Experience with the Malarial Treatment of General Paralysis in a State Institution," *American Journal of Psychiatry*, 84 (1928):715–27.

Jean H. Baker, *Mary Todd Lincoln, A Biography* (New York: W. W. Norton, 1987).

Philip R. Beard, "The Consumer Movement," chapter thirteen in Roy W. Menninger and John C. Nemiah, eds., *American Psychiatry after World War II, 1944– 1994* (Washington, D.C.: American Psychiatric Press, 2000).

Clifford W. Beers, *A Mind That Found Itself* (New York: Longmans, Green, 1908)

Allen E. Bergin and Sol L. Garfield, eds., *Handbook of Psychotherapy and Behavior Change* (New York: John Wiley and Sons, 1994).

David J. Bodenhamer and Robert G. Barrows, eds., *The Encyclopedia of Indianapolis* (Bloomington: Indiana University Press, 1994).

Thomas Neville Bonner, *Becoming a Physician: Medical Education in Britain, France, Germany, and the United States, 1750–1945* (Oxford University Press: New York, 1995).

Amariah Brigham, "Definition of Insanity—Nature of the Disease," *The American Journal of Insanity*, October 1844 (reprint, *Sesquicentennial Supplement to the American Journal of Psychiatry*, vol. 151, no. 6, June 1994):97–102.

Thomas J. Brown, *Dorothea Dix, New England Reformer* (Cambridge: Harvard University Press, 1998).

Catherine Clinton, *The Other Civil War: American Women in the Nineteenth Century* (New York: Hill and Wang, 1984).

_____and Christine Lunardini, *The Columbia Guide to American Women in the Nineteenth Century* (New York: Columbia University Press, 2000).

Eric T. Dean, Jr., *Shook over Hell: Post-Traumatic Stress, Vietnam, and the Civil War* (Cambridge: Harvard University Press, 1997).

John Demos, "The American Family in Past Time," *American Scholar*, 43(1974): 422–46.

Norman Dain, *Concepts of Insanity in the United States, 1789–1865* (New Brunswick, New Jersey: Rutgers University Press, 1964).

Pliny Earle, "The Curability of Insanity: A Statistical Study," *The American Journal of Insanity*, October 1885 (reprint, *Sesquicentennial Supplement to the American Journal of Psychiatry*, vol. 151, no. 6, June 1994):113–24.

Alan R. Felthouse and Anthony Hempel, "Combined Homicide-Suicides: A Review," *Journal of Forensic Sciences*, 40(1995):846–57.

Roger Finke and Rodney Stark, *The Churching of America, 1776–1900, Winners and Losers in Our Religious Economy* (New Brunswick, New Jersey: Rutgers University Press, 1992).

Glen O. Gabbard, "Empirical Evidence and Psychotherapy: A Growing Scientific Base," *American Journal of Psychiatry*, 158(2001):1–3.

Jeffrey L. Geller, "When Less Is More; When Less is Less," *Psychiatric Services*, 46(1995):1105.

_____, "The Last Half-Century of Psychiatric Services as Reflected in *Psychiatric Services*," *Psychiatric Services*, 51 (2000):41–67.

Gerald N. Grob, *The Mad among Us: a History of the Care of America's Mentally Ill* (New York: Free Press, 1994).

_____, "Psychiatry's Holy Grail: The Search for the Mechanism of Mental Diseases," *Bulletin of the History of Medicine*, 72(1998):189–219.

_____, "Mental Health Policy in Late Twentieth-Century America," chapter ten in Roy W. Menninger and John C. Nemiah, eds., *American Psychiatry after World War II, 1944–1994* (Washington, D.C.: American Psychiatric Press, 2000).

Shirley C. Guthrie, *Christian Doctrine* (Louisville, Kentucky: Westminster/ John Knox Press, 1994).

Joan Hoff, *Law, Gender, and Injustice: A Legal History of U.S. Women* (New York: New York University Press, 1993).

R. Douglas Hurt, *The Ohio Frontier: Crucible of the Old Northwest, 1720–1830* (Bloomington: Indiana University Press, 1996).

Paul E. Huston and Lillian M. Locher, "Manic-Depressive Psychosis: Course When Treated and Untreated with Electric Shock," *Archives of Neurology and Psychiatry*, 60(1948):37–48.

Steven E. Hyman and Eric J. Nestler, *The Molecular Foundations of Psychiatry* (Washington, D.C.: American Psychiatric Press,1993).

Kay Redfield Jamison, *Touched with Fire: Manic-Depressive Illness and the Artistic Temperament* (New York: Free Press, 1993).

_____, *Night Falls Fast: Understanding Suicide* (New York: Alfred A. Knopf, 1999).

Eric R. Kandel, "A New Intellectual Framework for Psychiatry," *American Journal of Psychiatry*, 155(1998):457–69.

R. C. Kessler et al., "Lifetime and 12-month Prevalence of DSM-III Psychiatric Disorders in the United States: Results from the National Comorbidity Survey," *Archives of General Psychiatry*, 51(1994):8–19.

Lucy Jane King, "A Brief History of Psychiatry: Millennia Past and Present, Part III," *Annals of Clinical Psychiatry*, 11(1999):99–107.

_____, "The Best Possible Means of Benefiting the Incurable: Walter Bruetsch and the Malaria Treatment of Paresis," *Annals of Clinical Psychiatry*, 12(2000): 197–203.

_____and Nancy L. Eckerman, "Creativity and Mood Disorders in Nineteenth Century Asylum Patients," *Journal of Medical Biography*, 9(2001):167–74.

Thomas S. Kirkbride, *On the Construction, Organization, and General Arrangements of Hospitals for the Insane with Some Remarks on Insanity and Its Treatment*(Philadelphia: J.B.Lippincott, 1880).

_____, "A Sketch of the History, Buildings, and Organization of the Pennsylvania Hospital for the Insane," *American Journal of Insanity*, October 1845 (reprint, *Sesquicentennial Supplement to the American Journal of Psychiatry*, vol. 151, no. 6, June, 1994):21–27.

S. J. Kleinberg, *Women in the United States, 1830–1945* (New Brunswick, New Jersey: Rutgers University Press, 1999).

Emil Kraepelin, *Manic-Depressive Insanity and Paranoia*, trans. R. Mary Barclay, ed. George M. Robertson(Edinburgh: E. and S. Livingstone, 1921).

H. Richard Lamb, "Deinstitutionalization and Public Policy," chapter eleven in Roy W. Menninger and John C. Nemiah, eds., *American Psychiatry after World War II, 1944—1994* (Washington, D.C.: American Psychiatric Press. 2000).

Kenneth M. Ludmerer, *Time to Heal: American Medical Education from the Turn of the Century to the Era of Managed Care* (Oxford: Oxford University Press, 1999).

Avram H. Mack, Leslie Forman, Rebekah Brown, and Allen Frances, "A Brief History of Psychiatric Classification," *Psychiatric Clinics of North America*, 17(1994): 515–23.

Jennie McCowen, *Women Physicians in Hospitals for the Insane*, Transactions Association for the Advancement of Women, October 1885, reprint (Buffalo: Peter Paul and Bro., Printers, 1886).

Roy W. Menninger and John C. Nemiah, eds., *American Psychiatry after World War II, 1944–1994* (Washington, D.C: American Psychiatric Press, 2000).

Mark E. Neely, Jr. and R. Gerald McMurtry, *The Insanity File: The Case of*

Mary Todd Lincoln (Carbondale: Southern Illinois University Press, 1986).

J. C. Norcross, ed., "A Roundtable on Psychotherapy Integration: Common Factors, Technical Eclecticism, and Psychotherapy Research," *Journal of Psychotherapy Practice and Research,* vol. 4, no. 3, 1995.

Lucy Ozarin, "As Others Saw Us . . . in 1875," *Psychiatric News,* March 17, 2000.

Joyce M. Ray and F. G. Gosling, "Historical Perspectives on the Treatment of Mental Illness in the United States" *Journal of Psychiatry and Law,* 10(1982):135–61.

Ruth Richards, "Conclusions: When Illness Yields Creativity," in Mark A. Runco and Ruth Richards, eds., *Eminent Creativity, Everyday Creativity, and Health,* (Greenwich, Connecticut: Ablex, 1997).

Eli Robins, *The Final Months: A Study of the Lives of 134 Persons Who Committed Suicide* (New York: Oxford University Press, 1981).

Lee N. Robins and Darrel A Regier, *Psychiatric Disorders in America, The Epidemiologic Catchment Area Study* (New York: Free Press, 1991)

D. L. Rosenhan, "On Being Sane in Insane Places," *Science,* 179(1974):250–8.

Mark A. Runco and Ruth Richards eds., *Eminent Creativity, Everyday Creativity, and Health* (Greenwich, Connecticut: Ablex,1997).

Barbara Sapinsley, *The Private War of Mrs. Packard* (New York: Paragon House, 1991).

David Satcher, *Mental Health: A Report of the Surgeon General* (Washington, D.C.:U. S. Public Health Service, December 1999).

Alan F. Schatzberg and Charles B. Nemeroff, eds., *Textbook of Psychopharmacology* (Washington, D.C.: American Psychiatric Press,1998).

Andrew Scull, Charlotte MacKenzie, Nicholas Hervey, *Masters of Bedlam: The Transformation of the Mad-Doctoring Trade* (Princeton, New Jersey: Princeton University Press, 1996).

Edward Shorter, *A History of Psychiatry: From the Era of the Asylum to the Age of Prozac* (New York: John Wiley and Sons, 1997).

R. S. Simons and F. H. Parker, *Railroads of Indiana* (Bloomington: Indiana University Press, 1997).

Jo Anne Sirey *et al.,* "Perceived Stigma as a Predictor of Treatment Discontinuation in Young and Older Outpatients with Depression," *American Journal of Psychiatry,* 158(2001):479–81.

Carroll Smith-Rosenberg, "The Hysterical Woman: Sex Roles and Role Conflict in Nineteenth–Century America," *Social Research,* 3(1972):652–78.

Michael H. Stone, *Healing the Mind: A History of Psychiatry from Antiquity to the Present* (New York: W .W. Norton, 1997).

W. Sutton, *The Western Book Trade: Cincinnati as a Nineteenth Century Publishing and Book Trade Center* (Columbus: Ohio State University Press, 1961).

Ann Taves, *Fits, Trances, and Visions, Experiencing Religion and Explaining Experience from Wesley to James* (Princeton, New Jersey: Princeton University

Press, 1999).

Paul Thagard, *How Scientists Explain Disease*(Princeton, New Jersey: Princeton University Press, 1999).

Emma Lou Thornbrough, *Indiana in the Civil War Era* (Indianapolis: Indiana Historical Bureau, Indiana Historical Society, 1965).

K. A. Tinsley, "Continuing Ties: Relations between Middle Class Parents and Their Children in Midwestern Families, 1870–1920," Ph.D. Dissertation (Madison: University of Wisconsin, 1995).

D. Hack Tuke, *The Insane in the United State and Canada* (London: H. K. Lewis, 1885).

Otto F. Wahl, *Telling Is Risky Business: Mental Health Consumers Confront Stigma* (New Brunswick, New Jersey: Rutgers University Press, 1999).

Mary Jane Ward, *The Snake Pit* (New York: New American Library, 1946).

John Harley Warner, *The Therapeutic Perspective: Medical Practice, Knowledge, and Identity in America, 1820–1885* (Princeton, New Jersey: Princeton University Press, 1997).

NOTES

Introduction

Max Bahr "A Hundred Years"; Central State Hospital closing, *Indianapolis Star*, October 1, 1993, December 2, 1994.

Chapter One

Indented quotations from Anna Agnew, *From under the Cloud* (Cincinnati: Robert Clarke and Company, 1886). All letters referred to were published in the *Indianapolis Herald* and signed Non Compos Mentis: August 1, 1885; November 18, 1885; January 16, 1886. The fourth letter to the *Herald* appears as a chapter in her book. Quotations of physicians and officials and data about the hospital are from *annual reports of the Indiana Hospital for the Insane* at the Indiana State Library, Indianapolis. Admission form, Indiana Hospital for the Insane: Central State Hospital, Admission Books, Female, Book 2, 321, Indiana State Archives, Indianapolis.

Brigham, "Definition of Insanity"; Clinton, The Other Civil War; Clinton and Lunardini, The Columbia Guide to American Women; Demos, "The American Family"; Dain, *Concepts of Insanity*, 6–7, postulated causes of insanity in the nineteenth century; Dean, *Shook over Hell*, Appendix C, Indiana Commitment Procedures; Earle, "The Curability of Insanity"; Grob, *The Mad AmongUs*; Kleinberg, *Women in the United States*; Kirkbride, On the Construction"; "A Sketch of the History"; Simons and Parker, *Railroads of Indiana*; Smith-Rosenberg, "The Hysterical Woman"; Warner, *The Therapeutic Perspective*, 64–65, temperament and illness.

Orpheus Everts: Obituaries, *Indiana Medical Journal*, 22(1903):37; *Journal of the Indiana State Medical Association*, 3(1910):76.

William W. Hester: George W. Warvelle, ed., A *Compendium of Freemasonry in Illinois*, vol. 1 (Chicago: Lewis Publishing Company, 1897), 608–9.

Chapter Two

See genealogy, below.
Hurt, The Ohio Frontier; Sutton, The Western Book Trade; Tinsley, "Continuing Ties."

Chapter Three

American Psychiatric Association, *Diagnostic and Statistical Manual of Mental Disorders, Fourth Edition, Text Revision* (Washington, D.C.: American Psychiatric Association, 2000), 356, 362, 821, 823; Dean, *Shook over Hell,* Civil War soldiers; Felthouse and Hempel, "Combined Homicide-Suicides"; Jamison, *Night Falls Fast;* Robins, *The Final Months.* See genealogy, below, for sources of information about the Agnews.

Chapter Four

Ellen Dwyer, "Central State Hospital," in Bodenhamer and Barrows, eds., *The Encyclopedia of Indianapolis,* 397–8.
Joseph Goodwin Rogers: Obituaries, *Journal of the Indiana State Medical Association,* 1(1908):205–6; *Indiana Medical Journal,* 26(1908):463.
John C. Walker: B. R. Sulgrave, *A History of Indianapolis and Marion County* (Philadelphia: L. H. Everts and Co., 1884), 294–6; Thornbrough, *Indiana in the Civil War Era,* 212–18; G. R. Tredway, *Democratic Opposition to the Lincoln Administration in Indiana* (Indianapolis: Indiana Historical Bureau, 1973), chapters 10, 11; G. W. H. Kemper, *A Medical History of the State of Indiana* (Chicago: American Medical Association Press, 1911), 352.

Chapter Five

Baker, *Mary Todd Lincoln,* tintype opposite 177 and accompanying text; Finke and Stark, *The Churching of America;* Guthrie, *Christian Doctrine,* 118–24; Taves, *Fits, Trances, and Visions;* Tuke, *The Insane in the United States.*

Chapter Six

Bonner, *Becoming a Physician,* 312–15, women physicians in the late nineteenth century; Brown, *Dorothea Dix,* 89, quotation; Hoff, *Law, Gender, and Injustice,* 152–61, Susan B. Anthony; McCowen, *Women Physicians in Hospitals for the Insane;* Ozarin, "As Others Saw Us", restraints in American asylums; Ray and Gosling, "Historical Perspectives," first three periods of reform; Scull et al., *Masters of Bedlam*, restraints in English asylums; Warner, *The Therapeutic Perspective*, 270–71, discovery of chloral hydrate.

Sheryl D. Vanderstel, "Calvin Fletcher," in Bodenhamer and Barrows, eds., *The Encyclopedia of Indianapolis*, 577-9.

W. B. Fletcher, "The Mystery of Insanity," *Indianapolis Herald*, August 22, 1885.

William Fletcher: R. French Stone, *Biography of Eminent American Physicians and Surgeons*, (Indianapolis: C. E. Hollenbeck Printer, 1898), 163–4; Obituary, *Indiana Medical Journal*, 25(1907):439–43; Rachael L. Drenovsky, "Humanity's Bonfire, William B. Fletcher, M.D., 1837–1907," *Traces of Indiana and Midwestern History*, spring 2001, 18–25.

Sarah Stockton: Obituaries, *Journal of the Indiana State Medical Association*, 17(1924):129; *Indianapolis Star*, March 14, 1924.

Andrew J. Thomas: Obituary, *Indiana Medical Journal*, 17(1898):36.

Chapter Seven

Geller, "When Less is More"; Satcher, *Mental Health*, preface; Sirey et al., "Perceived Stigma."

Hartford (Connecticut) *Courant*, October 11–15, 1998.

Wall Street Journal: Report, Health and Medicine: Can the System Be Fixed? "Model vs. Model, A Comparison of Countries' Health-care Systems," February 21, 2001.

Chapter Eight

See Genealogy below

Chapter Nine

Education: Bonner, *Becoming a Physician;* Ludmerer, *Time to Heal; Research in Mental Hospitals* (New York: The National Committee for Mental Hygiene, 1938), Central State Hospital, Indianapolis, 38.

Max Bahr: *Indianapolis Star*, February 27, 1938; *Indianapolis Times*, January 24, 1953; *Indiana Medical History Quarterly*, 7(1981):11; *Who's Who and What's What in Indiana* (1944), 747; *Indiana Today* (1942), 277, 378; Indiana Bibliography Series, Indiana State Library, Indianapolis, Indiana.

George Edenharter: R. French Stone, *Biography of Eminent American Physi-*

cians and Surgeons (Indianapolis: Carlan and Hollenbeck Publishers, 1894), 155–6; Jacob Piatt Dunn, Jr., *Greater Indianapolis: The History, the Industries, the Institutions, and the People of a City of Homes* (Chicago: Lewis Publishing Company, 1910), vol. 2, 975–8; Obituary, *Indianapolis News*, December 7, 1923.

Diagnosis: Baker, *Mary Todd Lincoln*; Grob, "Psychiatry's Holy Grail"; Kirkbride, *On the Contruction*, 249–50; Kandel, "A New Intellectual Framework for Psychiatry"; Kessler et al., "Lifetime and 12-month Prevalence"; Kraepelin, *Manic-Depressive Insanity*; Mack et al., "A Brief History"; Neely and McMurtry, *The Insanity File*; Richards, "Conclusions: When Illness Yields Creativity"; Rosenhan, "On Being Sane in Insane Places"; Sapinsley, *The Private War of Mrs. Packard*; Thagard, *How Scientists Explain Disease*, chapter two.

Psychopharmacology: Bahr and Bruetsch, "Two Years Experience"; Huston and Locher, *"Manic-Depressive Psychosis"*; Hyman and Nestler, *The Molecular Foundations of Psychiatry*; Schatzberg and Nemeroff, Textbook of Psychopharmacology; Shorter, *A History of Psychiatry*.

Walter Bruetsch: Charles A. Bonsett, "Walter Bruetsch," in Bodenhamer and Barrows, eds., *The Encyclopedia of Indianapolis*, 362; Bruetsch Papers, Box 1, Folder 16, p. 6, Indiana Medical History Museum, Indianapolis.

Psychosocial Therapies: Bergin and Garfield, *Handbook of Psychotherapy and Behavior Change*; Gabbard, "Empirical Evidence"; King, "A Brief History"; Norcross, "A Roundtable"; Stone, *Healing the Mind*.

Asylums in the Late Twentieth Century: Bachrach, "The State of the State Mental Hospital"; Beard, "The Consumer Movement"; Geller, "The Last Half-Century"; Grob, "Mental Health Policy"; Lamb, "Deinstitutionalization and Public Policy"; Menninger and Nemiah, *American Psychiatry after World War II, 1944–1994*; Robins and Regier, *Psychiatric Disorders in America*.

Dixmont State Hospital: *North Hills* (Pennsylvania) *News Record*, September 8, 1998, Dixmont State Hospital Collection, Box 2, Envelope #28, Library and Archives, Historical Society of Western Pennsylvania, Pittsburgh; *North Hills News Record*, January 30, 1999, www.nhnewsrecord.com; *Pittsburgh Tribune-Review*, September 18, 2000, www.triblive.com.

Indiana Hospital for the Insane: The *Indianapolis Star* reported in over forty articles about the closing of the hospital then called Central State Hospital. On October 1, 1993 it was reported that the governor had earlier ordered the hospital to be closed after a history of troubles and a series of patient deaths as well as allegations of employee abuse of patients.

Chapter Ten

Committee on Quality of Health Care in America, Institute of Medicine, *Crossing the Quality Chasm: A New Health Care System for the 21st Century*

(Washington, D.C.: National Academy Press, 2001), quotations from "Executive Summary," 1–23.

Dan Carpenter, "Mentally Ill Really Need These Drugs—Agreed?" *Indianapolis Star*, April 20, 2001.

Natalie Angier, "Together, In Sickness and In Health," *The New York Times Magazine*, May 6, 2001; Andrew Solomon, "A Cure for Poverty," *The New York Times Magazine*, May 6, 2001.

Satcher, "Organizing and Financing Mental Health Services," in *Mental Health*.

Genealogy

Origins, The Keyts and the Eskhams

Both Anna Keyt Agnew and her half-brother, Alonzo Keyt, wrote of their "old Dutch ancestry." Their grandfather John Keyt was born October 20, 1755, in Essex County, New Jersey. Their grandmother, his first wife, was Elizabeth Carter.

John Keyt was a private in the Revolutionary War. After the war he settled in the wilderness of the Old Northwest Territory along the Ohio River in what would soon become the seventeenth state, Ohio. Not long before he arrived there had been a battle in the area between Native Americans and settlers. A few miles to the southwest, speculators and merchants were settling the trade center of the Ohio Valley later called Cincinnati.

Nathan Keyt, John and Elizabeth's son and Anna and Alonzo Keyt's father, was born there in 1797. As a young man he was a teacher in the local school and the first postmaster of Moscow. He became a prominent citizen of Moscow holding several elective offices including that of mayor. He and a relative from his first marriage, to Alonzo's mother, were business partners as merchants, Keyt and Thrasher

Nathan Keyt's second wife, Martha Eskham, was Anna's mother. Martha was only sixteen in 1833 when she married Nathan, who was by then a widower more than twice her age. Martha, her parents, and four sisters had emigrated from England a little more than a decade before to take advantage of the unprecedented opportunity for immigrants in developing areas. Martha was marrying an established businessman active in community affairs. One of her sisters married Nathan Keyt's business partner, and the other sisters also married into local families.

Martha Eskham's youngest sister, Florilla, was born in 1822 after the family had settled in Ohio. Martha's mother had established friendship with a Mrs. Grant, who lived nearby. As an infant and young child, Florilla Eskham played with Mrs. Grant's son, Ulysses. Anna Agnew would later mention this and describe the Grant's home in one of her letters as "a quaint, old-fashioned, little house, with two front rooms and back kitchen," and noted that as a child she would not have thought that "so soon in the future that house would become famous as the birthplace of General Grant." The house stands today in Point Pleasant as Anna Agnew described it, now a national monument.

Clermont County, Ohio, 1980 (Batavia, Ohio: Clermont County Genealogical Society, 1981); Twylah Lemargie, Family Records, Clermont County Genealogical Society, Batavia, Ohio; J. L. Rockey, *History of Clermont County, Ohio, with Illustrations and Biographical Sketches of Its Prominent Men and Pioneers* (Philadelphia: Louis H. Everts, 1880); Alma Aicholz Smith, "Clermont County Deeds and Mortgages, 1791–1830, an Index," Clermont County Genealogical Society, Batavia, Ohio, 154; W. S. Stryker, ed., *The Revolutionary War*, (Trenton, New Jersey, 1872) 653; A. M. Whitt, *Clermont County, Ohio—1870: Atlas and History* (1870; reprint, Utica, Kentucky: McDowell Publications, 1985); all at Clermont County Public Library, Batavia, Ohio.

U.S. Census, Clermont County, Ohio, 1820, 1850, 1860.

Will of John Eskham, Anna Keyt Agnew's maternal grandfather, Probate Court Archives, Clermont County, Batavia, Ohio.

Nathan Keyte [Keyt] and Martha Eskum [Eskham] married October 8, 1833; George W. Irwin and Lida [Eliza] F. Keyt, May 27, 1867; Eugene L. Moore and Mary L. Keyt, March 31, 1868; David Agnew and Anna Keyt, April 13, 1870, Marriage Records, Probate Court Archives, Clermont County, Batavia, Ohio.

Frank B. Keyt, Anna Agnew's eldest brother, is listed as a law student in the U.S. Census, Clermont County, Ohio, 1860, and is mentioned as a lawyer in Batavia, the county seat of Clermont County, Ohio, in 1862. Rockey, *History of Clermont County, 139*.

Frank Keyt, died 1863; Mary Keyt Moore, died 1883; Martha Eskham Keyt, died 1897; and Nathan Keyt, died 1868; tombstones in the Moscow Cemetery. Missing details of the parent's now fragmented tombstones are in: Beech Forest Chapter, Daughters of the American Revolution, *Cemeteries in Clermont County, Ohio, 1952* (Evansville, Indiana: Unigraphic, Inc., 1980).

William H. H. Keyt, Anna Agnew's brother, U.S. Census, Covington, Kentucky, 1870, 1880:

Moores and Irwins: U.S. Census, Pittsburgh, Pennsylvania, 1880; Pittsburgh and Allegheny City Directories, 1868–1904, Genealogy Section, Pennsylvania Department, Carnegie Library, Pittsburgh, Pennsylvania.

Alonzo Keyt and his descendants: O. Juettner, *Daniel Drake and His Followers: Historical and Biographical Sketches, 1785–1909* (Cincinnati: Harvey Publishing Company, 1910); H. A. Kelly, *Cyclopedia of American Medical Biography* (Philadelphia: Saunders, 1912); Asa Brainerd Isham (Alonzo Keyt's son-in-law) and Mary Keyt Isham (Alonzo Keyt's granddaughter) *Cincinnati, the Queen City*, volume 3 (Cincinnati: S. J. Clarke Publishing Company, 1912). Alonzo Keyt's book on cardiology was published posthumously and edited by his son-in-law and son, both physicians. Alonzo T. Keyt, *Sphygmography and Cardiography, Physiological and Clinical*, A. B. Isham and M. H. Keyt, eds. (New York: G. P. Putnam's Sons, 1887).

Marriage and Children, the Agnews

Anna Agnew referred, with apparent sarcasm, to "the unspotted old Irish Presbyterian family into which I married." Agnews who settled in America did claim a proud heritage. Huguenot Agneaux had come to England with William the Conqueror in the eleventh century. Many Agnews settled in Scotland, where some became prominent citizens. Agnews, as would other Scots, became Presbyterian during the Protestant Reformation.

Some moved to Northern Ireland (Ulster) in the 1600s, encouraged by King James I who wanted Protestants to settle in that Catholic land. Their fortunes were to fluctuate according to the religious perspectives of rulers of England and conflicts with their Irish Catholic neighbors. In 1718 a great migration from Ulster to America began. Religious conflict, persecution of dissenters by the Church of England, drought in Ireland in 1714 to 1719, a decimation of the wool trade in which they were engaged due to a disease among sheep, a smallpox epidemic in 1718, and several bad harvests in the 1720s contributed to their leaving for America.

Many came to Philadelphia to enjoy religious freedom and to participate in the busy economy. During the course of the eighteenth century, some Agnews and their relatives became ministers, lawyers, doctors, professors, or prosperous businessmen in Philadelphia. By the time the Declaration of Independence was signed, one-sixth of the population of the thirteen colonies was Scottish or Scotch Irish Presbyterians.

Mary Virginia Agnew, *The Book of the Agnews* (Philadelphia: J. E. Caldwell and Co., 1926); William Forbes Marshall, *Ulster Sails West* (Belfast: The Quota Press, 1943); Ruth L. Mine, "Gibson Agnew, His Family and Descendents," Genealogy Department, Allen County Public Library, Fort Wayne, Indiana.

David Agnew's parents did not arrive until the early nineteenth century and were likely laborers or farmers according to immigration records and histories of the time. He was born in Philadelphia in 1843. U.S. Census, Vincennes, Indiana, 1880; Graves Registration Card, Adjutant General's Department, Archives/Library Division, Ohio Historical Center, Columbus.

Corporal David Agnew, 98th Ohio Infantry, Veterans Records, National Archives, Washington, D.C.; 98th Ohio Infantry: F. H. Dyer, *A Compendium of the War of the Rebellion* (1909; reprint, New York: Thomas Yoseloff, 1959) volume 1, 211, 450; volume 2, 154; E. B. Long and B. Long, *The Civil War Day by Day: An Almanac, 1861–1865* (Garden City, New York: Doubleday and Company, 1971).

David Agnew worked as a clerk at the Ohio and Mississippi Railroad from

1868 to1871. In 1868 through 1870 his home addresses indicate that he was a boarder. He had a new address in 1871, probably David and Anna Agnew's first residence: City Directories, Cincinnati, Ohio.

David Agnew, Nathan age 9, William age 7, David age 5, a housekeeper, and Anna "insane" [she had already been hospitalized]: U.S. Census, Vincennes, Indiana, 1880. All census records indicate that Nathan was born in Ohio and that William and David were both born in Indiana. They were probably born in Seymour, although David might have been born in Vincennes. There are no birth records for Indiana in the 1870s. *History of Jackson County, Indiana* (Chicago: Brant and Fuller, 1886); L. W. Noblitt, *The Composite History of Jackson County, Indiana* (Paducah, Kentucky: Turner Publishing Company, 1991).

David Agnew: Personal property tax records, 1877, 1878, 1880, 1881, and 1882, Knox County Records, Vincennes, Indiana. City Directories, Vincennes, 1880, Lewis Historical Library, Vincennes University, and 1881, Knox County Library, Historical Collection; *Historical Sketches of Old Vincennes, its institutions and churches* (Vincennes, 1903), 479, Indiana State Library, Indianapolis; *History of Knox and Daviess Counties, Indiana* (Chicago: Goodspeed Publishing Company, 1886).

"A child of David Agnew, clerk in the Auditor's Office on the O. and M. road, fell out of a tree one day last week and broke both of his arms . . . Mr. Agnew has lately located at Walkertown" [a section of Aurora, Indiana] "News from Aurora," *Lawrenceburg* (Indiana) *Register*, May 3, 1883; State vs. David Agnew, desertion of wife, *nolle prosequi*; "Court Reports," *Lawrenceburg Register*, September 3 and November 26, 1885; *History of Dearborn and Ohio Counties* (1885; reprint, Evansville: Wipporwill Publications, 1986).

David Agnew and his three sons, their addresses, and where they worked (not all the sons are listed in all the directories): City Directories, Cincinnati, Ohio, 1886-1897.

Youngest son David F. Agnew, railroad clerk: Cincinnati City Directory, 1892. When Anna Agnew entered Dixmont Hospital in 1894, she was recorded as having three sons, the youngest in his nineteenth year. That would have been David.

Second son William N. Agnew, "moved to Louisville": Cincinnati City Directory, 1895. He is named in City Directories, Louisville, Kentucky, 1897–99. David Agnew's military grave record, 1911, lists William as next of kin, then living in New Jersey.

Eldest son Nathan Keyt Agnew: City Directories, Evansville, Indiana, 1895–1898; J. P. Elliott, *A History of Evansville and Vanderburgh County, Indiana* (Evansville: Keller Printing Company, 1897), 285; Marriage License, records of Vanderburgh County, Genealogy Section, Indiana State Library, Indianapolis; society column, *Evansville Courier*, October 20, 1901.

David Agnew living in Cincinnati and working for the Cincinnati, Hamilton, and Dayton Railroad: Cincinnati City Directories, 1900–1909; *The Story of the*

Baltimore and Ohio Railroad, 1827–1927 (New York: G. P. Putnam's Sons, 1928) vol. 2, 258–9; Corporal David Agnew, Company I, 98th Ohio Infantry, tombstone, Dayton National Cemetery, Dayton, Ohio.

Anna, Divorced

U.S. Census, Pittsburgh, Pennsylvania, 1880; Pittsburgh and Allegheny City Directories, 1868–1904, Genealogy Section, Pennsylvania Department, Carnegie Library, Pittsburgh; *Pennsylvania Historical Review, Gazetteer, Post-office, Express, and Telegraph Guide* (New York: Historical Publishing Company, 1886), 112.

City Directories for Pittsburgh in the early 1870s, 1880s, and 1890s list George W. Irwin's home address in Pittsburgh. In the early 1900s, his local office address is at the chemical company, but his home address is "Brooklyn, New York." U.S. Census, Borough of Brooklyn, New York, 1900, lists a George W. Irwin, age 55, born Ohio, whose wife of three years was named Mary. She had no children. The daughters living with them have the same names and birth dates as daughters previously listed with George W. and Lida Keyt Irwin in the 1880 Pittsburgh Census and were born in Pennsylvania. In all probability, Lida Keyt Irwin had died in the 1890s, and George W. Irwin had remarried. He died March 1, 1913, age 68: Obituary, *Pittsburgh Gazette*, March 5, 1913, Pennsylvania Department, Carnegie Library, Pittsburgh.

Summary, Anna Agnew's Record, Admission Book, 1892–1917; Patient History Book, 1893–1894, Dixmont State Hospital, supplied by William Penn Memorial Museum and Archives, Pennsylvania Historical and Museum Commission, Harrisburg. (Medical information deleted in accordance with Pennsylvania statute); Dixmont State Hospital Collection, Library and Archives, Historical Society of Western Pennsylvania, Pittsburgh; Anna Agnew, aged 64 and 74, respectively, born Ohio, patient at Dixmont State Hospital: U.S. Census, Pittsburgh and Allegheny County, 1900, 1910.

Index